Your Body Is Not A Car

The Secrets for Good Health
Based on Traditional Chinese Medicine

by Pindy Yin-Ping Wong, L. Ac., O. M. D., Ph. D.
and Hoenie Wai-Shun Luk, Ph. D.

Almond Publishing
P. O. Box 573
Petaluma, CA 94953

Note to readers:

This book is intended to document a healing tradition and, as such, is not a substitute for professional medical advice or services to the individual readers. While every effort has been made to ensure that the information presented in this book is accurate and complete, neither the authors nor the publisher shall be responsible for any loss, injury or damage that may result from any information contained in this book.

Almond Publishing
P. O. Box 573
Petaluma, CA 94953
http://www.almondpublishing.com

Copyright © 2008 by Pindy Wong and Hoenie Luk

All rights reserved.
No part of this book shall be reproduced in any form without permission by the authors.

Wong, Pindy and Luk, Hoenie
Your Body Is Not A Car:
The Secrets for Good Health Based on Traditional Chinese Medicine

ISBN 978-0-9777314-0-4
Library of Congress Control Number: 2008931685

Dedicated to

all our patients,

past, present and future,

from whom we have learned so much of what is written in this book.

Contents

About the authors..........ix

CHAPTER 1
THE ESSENCE OF GOOD HEALTH..........1

Sect. 1-1: Why is your body not a car?..........1

Sect. 1-2: The working principle of diseases according to traditional Chinese medicine..........4

Sect. 1-3: The goal of this book..........7

Sect. 1-4: What is good health?..........9

Sect. 1-5: The Taoist theory of Yin and Yang..........11

Sect. 1-6: The body's fuel tank as a bank account: vital substance and vital force..........14

Sect. 1-7: The body machine as a steam engine: chi..........16

Sect. 1-8: The human body as a self-healing machine..........18

Sect. 1-9: Once again, what is good health and what are good health habits?..........22

CHAPTER 2
MAXIMIZING VITAL SUBSTANCE..........25

Sect. 2-1: The downward spiral of poor digestion..........26

Sect. 2-2: A tour of the digestive process: the beginning..........28

Sect. 2-3: Digestion in the stomach..........31

Sect. 2-4: Digestion and absorption in the small intestine..........34

Sect. 2-5: Elimination in the large intestine..........38

Sect. 2-6: TCM concepts of digestion..........40

Sect. 2-7: Eating well-balanced meals..........42

Sect. 2-8: Eating fruit after lunch and dinner..........47

Sect. 2-9: Accompanying each meal with a hot fluid..........48

Sect. 2-10: Foods to avoid..........50
    (a) Cold drinks and foods..........50
    (b) Raw foods..........52
    (c) Direct-fire and deep-fried foods..........53
    (d) Spicy foods..........54
    (e) Garlic..........56
    (f) Overly sweetened foods..........57
    (g) Supplements..........59
    (h) Stimulants — caffeine, alcohol, cigarette and recreational drugs..........60

Sect. 2-11: Regular mealtimes..........62
    (a) Breakfast..........65
    (b) Lunch..........66
    (c) Dinner..........67

Sect. 2-12: Proper cooking methods..........68
    (a) Grains..........71
    (b) Vegetables..........71
    (c) Meat, poultry and fish..........73

Sect. 2-13: Practical tips for eating out..........76

CHAPTER 3
CONSERVING VITAL FORCE..........81

Sect. 3-1: The global consequences of energy debt..........81
    (a) Chronic fatigue..........84
    (b) Digestive problems..........85
    (c) Insomnia..........86
    (d) Hot flashes (night sweats)..........87
    (e) Weak immune system..........88
    (f) Muscle and tendon injuries..........88
    (g) Negative mental and emotional states..........89
    (h) Return of old symptoms..........90
    (i) Weight gain..........90

Sect. 3-2: Activities that interfere with resting..........92
    (a) Nighttime activity..........92
    (b) Inadequate breaks..........95

Sect. 3-3: Over-exercising..........95

Sect. 3-4: Intensified mental and emotional states..........99

Sect. 3-5: Unnecessary heat loss..........102

    (a) Weather conditions..........103

    (b) Direct contact..........106

    (c) Breathing dry or damp air 106

    (d) Faulty washing habits..........107

    (e) Highly-contrasting indoor and outdoor temperatures..........109

    (f) Eating cold food and drinks..........111

CHAPTER 4
ENHANCING CHI..........113

Sect. 4-1: The dilemma with regular exercises..........113

Sect. 4-2: Non-movement-style chi gong..........116

Sect. 4-3: Moving-style and martial-art-style chi gong..........121

Sect. 4-4: Chi-enhancing therapies..........124

    (a) Acupressure..........124

    (b) Reflexology..........125

Sect. 4-5: Practicing chi-enhancing techniques..........127

CHAPTER 5
PROMOTING SELF-HEALING..........129

Sect. 5-1: Your other job starts at 10:30 P.M...........130

Sect. 5-2: The meridian clock of self-regeneration..........132

Sect. 5-3: Why the liver holds the key to all diseases..........133

    (a) On digestive system..........134

    (b) On excretory system..........135

    (c) On nervous system..........136

    (d) On endocrine and reproductive systems..........137

    (e) On immune system..........137

    (f) On circulatory system..........138

Sect. 5-4: Liver and gall bladder have the most hazardous job of all..........140
    (a) Extreme blood..........140
    (b) Food-borne pathogens..........141
    (c) Natural and artificial toxins..........141
    (d) Reactive oxygen species..........141
    (e) Gallstones..........142
    (f) Blood congestion..........143
    (g) Emotional stress..........144
Sect. 5-5: The TCM strategy for a healthy liver..........145
Sect. 5-6: Promoting good-quality sleep..........148
Sect. 5-7: Recharging during the day..........150
    (a) Regular breaks..........151
    (b) Lunch break..........151
    (c) Overtime work..........152
Sect. 5-8: Recharging throughout the year..........153
    (a) Winter dormancy..........153
    (b) Vacations..........154
    (c) Hobbies..........154

CHAPTER 6
GOOD HEALTH HABITS..........157

Sect. 6-1: The task ahead..........157
Sect. 6-2: The complete list of good health habits..........158

INDEX..........167

About the authors

Pindy Wong, L. Ac., O. M. D., Ph. D., began her clinical training in traditional Chinese medicine (TCM) in Hong Kong under the tutelage of her grandfather at the age of nine and, in the process, she earned the nickname "Angel Fingers" for her ability to heal. For the next 12 years, she went on to work as apprentice under twelve other TCM specialists throughout Hong Kong and China.

Ms. Wong began practicing TCM in San Francisco and San Rafael, California, in mid 1980's. In addition to becoming a licensed acupuncturist (L. Ac.) in California, she obtained further clinical training at Guangxi College of Traditional Chinese Medicine in China. In the U. S., she broadened her scope of knowledge through a series of academic training, earning several degrees including:
- Doctor in Oriental Medicine (O. M. D.)
- Ph. D. in Oriental Medicine
- Fellowship in Orthopedics & Traumatology

Even today, Ms. Wong is keenly interested in Western herbalism as a way to supplement her arsenal of Chinese herbs.

Ms. Wong is a strong advocate of using proper food and cooking for the maintenance of health. Much of the cooking techniques she uses are the result of advanced training in commercial and home-style cooking and pastries (in both Western and Eastern cuisines) at Maria's Culinary Arts School in Hong Kong.

In 1995, Ms. Wong established her current private practice in Petaluma, California, where she continues to offer TCM threrapies including acupuncture, acupressure, reflexology, dietary instruction, herbal zone therapy, herbal thread moxibustion, herbal cupping and herbal medicine.

Hoenie Luk, Ph. D., is well-versed in modern biology as he earned his B.A. degree in Zoology from University of California at Berkeley (UCB) and, subsequently, his Ph. D. degree in Biomedical Sciences from University of California at San Francisco (UCSF), where he did laboratory research on peripheral nerve regeneration.

Many people know him as a teacher as he spent many years teaching biology in high schools, college and private tutoring, as well as histology (the study of tissues) in pharmacy school and medical school.

As the son of Pindy Wong, he has been a long-time user of traditional Chinese medicine and is very familiar with the healthy living habits advocated by Pindy. His current interest is focused in medicinal plants and California native plants, as he leads frequent plant walks in the San Francisco Bay Area for San Francisco Homeschoolers and California Native Plant Society.

CHAPTER 1
THE ESSENCE OF GOOD HEALTH

Sect. 1-1: Why is your body not a car?

Sect. 1-2: The working principle of diseases according to traditional Chinese medicine

Sect 1-3: The goal of this book

Sect 1-4: What is good health?

Sect 1-5: The Taoist theory of Yin and Yang

Sect 1-6: The body's fuel tank as a bank account: vital substance and vital force

Sect 1-7: The body machine as a steam engine: chi

Sect 1-8: The human body as a self-healing machine

Sect 1-9: Once again, what is good health and what are good health habits?

Sect. 1-1: Why is your body not a car?

We often compare the human body with a finely-tuned machine, such as a car. After all, the body is consisted of many complex organ systems, just as a car is consisted of many mechanical and electrical systems, all working in harmony to produce useful work. The body also shares many characteristics with a car — they both consume fuel, they both exercise, they both break down once in a while and need to be repaired, they both age and eventually fail completely. If the body is so similar to a car, what is wrong with thinking of the body as a car?

A high performance car — powerful, complicated and intriguing, just like the human body.

For over a decade, I (P.W.) have been practicing acupuncture and traditional Chinese medicine (TCM) at a clinic in the city of Petaluma (northern California) and the vast majority of my patients are Westerners (i.e. non-Asians). They come to see me for a wide variety of health problems, ranging from chronic diseases like insomnia, premenstrual syndromes, indigestion, depression, premature menopause, chronic fatigue and tendinitis, to acute diseases such as stomach disorder, frontal headache, bladder infection, hives, rashes, diarrhea, Bell's Palsy, ovarian cysts, anxiety, non-functional behavior and proneness to injury. If this list impresses you as rather lengthy, it should also impress you that the conditions listed are all very common among people living in today's modern society.

Here is an interesting question: why are these diseases so common nowadays? To be sure, modern life, with accelerating pace and competition, has become more and more stressful. As we become more occupied with things revolving around us, sometimes, without our full awareness, we begin to neglect our own well being. That's when we begin to treat our body as a car and problems begin to happen.

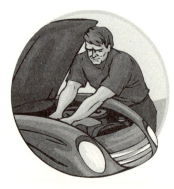

We leave all our car problems for the mechanic, trusting that he can always get them fixed. Can we do the same with our health problems?

What did you do when your car broke down? I took mine to a garage and told the mechanic to fix it. When the car was fixed, the mechanic called me, I paid the bill, grumbled about the expensive cost, and drove my car away. Funny enough, I was never seriously involved in any part of the whole process, except the money exchange.

True, sometimes the mechanic would mention to me the problem of my car, but with a line of customers behind me, he was always in a hurry. His explanation was always terse and barely comprehensible by a mere driver like me. As I probably would not understand complicated machines anyway, I was usually content to know just which parts had been fixed and merrily get back on the road. Fortunately, that seems to work fine for my car.

But perhaps because it works so well for their cars, many people take the same "hands-off" approach in handling their bodies when they become sick — they expect to be swiftly healed with only minimal involvement. Sometimes, they go to their doctors and expect to be given a magical pill or operation that will quickly cure their illnesses. Other times, they seek out quick fixes which saturated the commercial market for treating bodily inconveniences. Can't stay awake? Drink a cup of coffee. Can't fall asleep? Reach for the sleeping pill. Feeling fatigue? Take some stimulant. Feeling lousy? Have a few (or more) drinks of alcohol. Feeling hungry? Grab a candy bar. Having a headache? Pop some painkillers. What is wrong with this scenario?

What's wrong is that the body is really not a car and should never be treated like a car. Realistically, instant fixes never work for more than a short while — they make you feel better by masking the symptoms but the root causes remain untouched. Moreover drugs intended to be quick fixes often bring with them undesirable side-effects when used too often, which means that the body will feel even worse once the short-lived effect wears out.

Here are the two main reasons why quick fixes only work on your car but not on your body. First, the body cannot be fixed by replacing defective parts like a mechanic does with a car. True, modern medicine allows us to transplant heart, lung, kidney, liver, skin, cornea and a whole variety of body parts, but these expensive and risky procedures are not available except for the most desperate situations. As for replacement hip, replacement joint, artificial heart, artificial limbs and prosthetic teeth, etc., they are but inferior substitute of the real things, both functionally and aesthetically. You won't get your hip replaced and proclaim, "This looks as good as new!" as you would say after replacing the windshield of your car.

Second, your body, unlike your car, stays with you for your whole life. For our car, we can always console ourselves that we can buy a new one when it starts having too many mechanical

> First, the body cannot be fixed by replacing defective parts like a mechanic does with a car.... Second, your body, unlike your car, stays with you for your whole life.

failures. But can you change to a new body every four years to keep yourself in good performance?

Since you have to keep using the same body, quick fixes, which do not eliminate the root causes of health problems, simply allow those health problems to accumulate. By the time you reach middle age (just over 40), you, the owner of the body, will begin to feel the accumulative impact of the damages — but you still have another forty years to go — and no way out of your body.

In short, you cannot repair the body as casually as you take your car to the mechanic. If you do, the problems will come back to haunt you just when you realize you are stuck in your old wreck. I hope you are now convinced that your body is indeed different from a car and that you should treat your body more seriously than you would treat your car. If you have achieved this new level of enlightenment, you are on the right track to good health. But what exactly do we need to know to properly care for our bodies?

Sect. 1-2: The working principle of diseases according to traditional Chinese medicine

At the minimum, you need to know the most fundamental theory of why we become sick. There are different theories of diseases in different cultures — some attribute diseases to evil spirits, some to a person's misfortune, and some to tiny, invisible, disease-causing agents called germs (hence, the "germ theory"). But in Chinese medicine, the working principle of diseases, in its simplest form, states that a patient's condition is not purely the result of random and uncontrollable events, but rather, directly or indirectly, the result of the way he carries out life with his body. In other words, the way you treat your body

> In TCM, the working principle of diseases states that a patient's condition is, directly or indirectly, the result of the way he carries out life with his body.

influences the chance of you "catching" diseases and, if you do catch one, the chance of recovering from it.

For those of us who are parents, this is just common sense that we teach to our children every day. For example, we teach our children that they will get stomach ache if they put dirty food in their mouths and they will catch cold if they don't put on a jacket when they go outside when it is cold. The golden rule to good health is always the same — you will get sick if you do not treat your body right.

But what if I tell you that this principle is a lot more encompassing than you think? That it is applicable even to adult diseases, such as those listed earlier in the long catalog of modern-day ailments (second paragraph of Sect. 1-1)? That will be a surprise to many people. In fact, according to Chinese medicine, every disease in that list, as well as many others that we regard as idiopathic (meaning diseases that have no known cause), are directly or indirectly influenced by how we carry out our lives.

Of course, it is not obvious, at this point, how our own action can influence the chance we contract, say, ovarian cysts or gallstones — we will tackle that in the next several chapters of this book. But let me point out how empowering this working principle is in terms of the healing of a patient.

To illustrate this point, let me use the example of influenza, also known as the common flu. In the 18th century, people in Italy believed that influenza was caused by the "influence" of stars and planets — which was why they named the disease influenza, derived from the Latin word "influentia". It was not until 1933 when modern science finally discovered that influenza is caused by several types of fast-mutating RNA-containing virus now called influenza virus. Influenza virus type A is the cause of the majority of cases of common flu today.

Why do you think she got the flu?

Let's imagine it is now year 1900 and, as in the case of many other idiopathic diseases, science has not yet discovered the cause of common flu. Does that mean we are totally helpless against the flu and have to silently suffer from the disease?

Speaking from personal experience, one of the authors of this book (H.L.) used to be a high-school biology teacher. Every year from November to April, as the weather drastically changed, he would have many students in various stages of flu, coughing and blowing their noses in the crowded classroom. Being relatively healthy and physically active himself, fortunately, he was able to stay healthy most of the time.

However he did fall ill from contracting the flu once or twice a year. He then noticed that, when he did fall ill, it usually happened within one week after staying up late for several nights in a row in order to catch up with all the school work. Apparently, not having sufficient sleep could reduce the body's resistance against the flu.

Thus, in order to avoid contracting the flu, he consciously forced himself to go to bed on time to get at least seven hours of sleep, especially during those months when the flu was active. For the most part, he succeeded in keeping the flu at bay simply by strictly regulating his work and rest pattern. Even if he did get the flu, some Chinese herbs and acupuncture was all he needed to put himself back in action.

> While we, as individuals, may have no control over the seasonal outbreak of viruses, we do have much greater control on our own life habit — and, consequently, the destiny of our health.

This example illustrates several important points. Although it is true that the influenza virus is the direct cause of the flu disease, we don't necessarily contract the disease just because the virus exists around us. From the perspective of a patient, it appears that an insufficient amount of sleep is what causes the disease. Here, the patient's life habit is an indirect cause of the disease, not a direct one — but a real cause nonetheless. The most important point, however, is that while we, as individuals, may have no control over the seasonal outbreak of viruses, we do have much greater control on our own life habit — and, consequently, on the destiny of our health.

This, in turn, is the reason why a patient must actively participate in the healing process by adjusting their health habits — that means to not treat your body absentmindedly like a car. Clearly, conducting your everyday life with the proper health habits is the key to good health. But how do you know what good health habits are? The answer to this question, it turns out, is not at all obvious or straightforward. In fact, this complicated topic is what this book is all about.

Sect. 1-3: The goal of this book

This book is about how we can use good health habits to promote good health and to heal ourselves from sickness. But before I continue with the discussion of health habits, I want to take a moment to explain why I decided to write this book and what I hope to accomplish with it.

Every day at my clinic of traditional Chinese medicine (TCM), I see patients with a wide range of health problems. As you can now understand, besides giving out therapies and herbs, the most important part of my job is to educate my patients the proper health habits necessary to facilitate their recovery. This obviously involves the explaining of TCM concepts, which presented me with two challenges that eventually prompted me to write this book.

The first challenge is the limited time available at the clinical setting. While I spend an average of 30 minutes face-to-face with each patient, I barely have enough time to gleam through the most essential ideas and have to skip through much of the details. As you will soon see, there are so many misconceptions of health that I need to discuss that I could not adequately impress

Time is limited in a typical visit of an acupuncturist's office.

my patients on how much of their health is strictly under their own control.

The second challenge is the fact that TCM principles are the culmination of the Eastern way of living which most Westerners find unfamiliar, counterintuitive, or even downright bizarre, both in philosophy and in practice. Naturally, I need to take extra effort to bridge the linguistic and cultural gaps while my patients need extra time to gradually digest and absorb the information. Furthermore, these concepts need to be re-explained and revisited by the patients as they progress in their healing process.

I finally decided that the best way to meet both challenges is to put this large volume of knowledge in print so that you can take it home and learn it at a pace you feel most comfortable with. You can return and refer to this book from time to time as you experience the changes in your health conditions. With this book, you will learn systematically the same vital knowledge which I impart to my patients at my clinic. You will then be able to assist in enhancing the therapies you receive and continue to enjoy a trouble-free body after the therapies.

As you join the rank of healthy people, this book offers a path to prevent sickness, stay healthy and look for the body's signals which precede potential diseases. It is my hope that when you know the proper way to live within your body, you will enjoy a smooth-running machine without major breakdown.

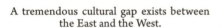
A tremendous cultural gap exists between the East and the West.

Sect. 1-4: What is good health?

Let us return to the question of what health habits are good health habits. Obviously, good health habits are health habits that lead to good health. So perhaps a more fundamental question to ask is this: what exactly do we mean by "good health"? How do you know if someone is in good health, anyway?

Just when you think the answer is obvious, many people in the modern society carry misconceptions of what good health actually means. Ask several people around you and you will hear several different interpretations of the term "good health".

One conventional idea of good health is based on the measurement of some athletic or work performance. Some people consider themselves to be in good shape, "if I can bench press 200 pounds", or "if I can do one hundred sit-ups", or "if I can run five miles every day" or "if I can work overtime for days in a row."

Another conventional idea of good health, favored by those conscious of their body images, is based on the comparison with a certain ideal body shape. Many people consider themselves in good health "if I have a flat belly", or "if I am not overweight", or "if I have a slim 36-23-36 figure", or "if I have a low BMI (body fat index)", or "if I have bulky muscles", or "if I have the body of Mr. Galaxy".

Yet another common interpretation of "good health", favored by the less ambitious, is the equivalence of "the absence of diseases". Therefore, if you are sneezing, coughing, aching, nauseating, collapsing, paralyzed, injured, lethargic or otherwise feeling uncomfortable, you are not in good health. But if you feel fine, then you are enjoying good health.

Unfortunately, all of the above interpretations of "good health" are problematic since they are all superficial and insufficient,

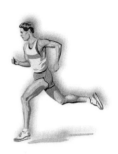
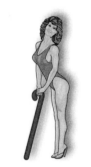
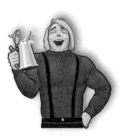

An athlete in top performance, a model with beautiful figure and a man feeling great: can you tell which of the three are in good health?

sometimes even misleading. For example, competitive body builders, considered to be the ultimate of healthy bodies by many, have to press their bodies to "tiptop" shape prior to competitions with a highly unbalanced diet and a strenuous training regiment for a prolonged period of time. While appearing strong on stage, body builders often admit to be feeling hurt and vulnerable inside, nearing the verge of collapse. This is a feeling we hardly associate with good health.

Take another example: some people run five miles every day after work because they believe that they must do the exercise to stay healthy and that they are healthy as long as they can perform the exercise. In reality, this may or may not be true depending on his work load and stress level during the day. I have treated many patients with high-paying but stressful job who were totally spent by the end of the work day but still dragged themselves to the gym to perform their daily prescribed exercise. Little did they know that they had become very prone to injury and suffered from chronic fatigue due to over-exhaustion.

What about the idea of "good health" as "the lack of diseases"? The trouble with this interpretation is that our feeling at the moment may not reveal certain underlying problems with our body until some unexpected events occur. Many first-time patients of heart attack, diabetes, high blood pressure and cancer are not aware of any potential problems with their bodies until one fateful day when something bad happens. Sometimes a person is not aware that his body has become very vulnerable to diseases until he contracts the mundane flu or cold and find that he has trouble recovering for a prolonged period of time.

> It should be amply clear that the conventional ideas of "good health" do not serve us well — they lead us to think that we are in good health while, in fact, we are not, or vice versa.

In addition, a lot of feelings of discomfort are not serious enough to be diagnosed as a disease by physicians, medical instruments or laboratory tests. What about the sore on the lower back which refuses to go away? What about waking up at 3 o'clock in the morning and not being able to go back to sleep? What about having to go to the bathroom three or four times every night during sleep? What about frequently falling asleep on the job? What about that foul-smelling breath? What about a very light amount of menstrual flow? What about that lingering cough? Granted, these could be signs that alert us of serious diseases ahead but, without knowing their significance, we often dismiss them as minor inconveniences and fall into the illusion that we are enjoying good health — until a real disease happens to us.

I think it should be amply clear by now that the conventional ideas of "good health" do not serve us well — they lead us to think that we are in good health while, in fact, we are not, or vice versa. In the following sections, I will introduce to you a more comprehensive and holistic interpretation of "good health" based on the principles of traditional Chinese medicine. It encompasses multiple aspects of our body functions and take into account the body's resistance against diseases. But to give you a full account of the story, we have to go back to the origin of the Taoist (道教) philosophy, 2400 years ago in ancient China.

Sect. 1-5: The Taoist theory of Yin and Yang

During the Warring States period (戰國時代) of China in the Eastern Zhou Dynasty (東周) around the 4th century B. C., China was divided into tens of rivaling states, each with its own "emperor" and government system. As each state struggled to be more powerful than its neighbors in order to conquer and to avoid being conquered, there were frequent debates among the academics over what political philosophies should be adopted to better govern the people and nurture a strong society. This is not unlike the

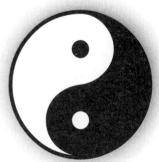

The yin-yang symbol consists of a bright top half (the sky) and a dark bottom half (the earth) — two opposite but inseparable forces that combine to form the complete natural world.

kind of discussions among present-day political science students over different social systems such as capitalism, democracy, socialism and communism, etc.

Apparently these political philosophers were very influential and highly respected — so much so that the "emperors" of many states customarily invited and patronized them for advice. Among the philosophers, the most famous one has to be Confucius (孔子), whose system of philosophy became known as Confucianism (孔教), which many historians regard as the foundation of morality in Chinese and Japanese cultures. But developed at about the same time and often operating in opposite direction as Confucianism was another system of philosophy which eventually found its way into the foundation of traditional Chinese medicine — Taoism (道教) (sometimes spelled Daoism, by mandarin phonics).

Laozi (老子), the original contributor of Taoist philosophy, rode his water buffalo to the western frontier of China in order to live as a hermit.

The word Tao (道) literally means "the way" and it refers to the way of nature, implying that humans should live by the principles with which nature has been operating in harmony for countless eons. Among the most fundamental of these principles was the observation that, invariably, every entity in nature consists of two forces that display the opposite properties of each other. For example, a day is made of day time and night time — the previous is bright and warm while the latter is dark and cool. The climate, in the perspective of a growing plant, is a combination of sunshine and rain — the previous is hot and dry while the latter is cool and wet. In the life cycle of a species, there are birth and death — the previous increases while the latter decreases the population. Similarly, you can easily come up with countless other examples.

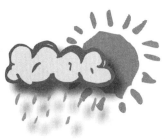

Too much rain, we get flooding. Too much sun, we get drought. Life on Earth depends on a balance between rain (yin) and sun (yang).

But not only that, Taoist philosophers also observed that, in nature, the quality or wholeness of an entity depends on the intricate balance of its two opposite forces. If, in a particular year, there is too much sun but too little rain, the land will experience scorching drought; but if there is too much rain and too little sun, the land will experience torrential flooding. In either case, the crops will fail and the harvest will suffer that year. In order for the climate to achieve wholeness, there must be a union of the two opposite forces, sunshine and rainfall, in a total and balanced package.

For a population, if there are too many births compared to deaths, there will be overpopulation, shortage of resources and, eventually, starvation will result; in the contrary, if there are too many deaths compared to births, there will be an aging of the population, a lack of regeneration of young individuals, and eventually the species will become extinct. In order for a population to stay healthy and vivacious, there must be a proper balance of the two opposite forces, birth and death.

> In nature, the quality or wholeness of an entity depends on the intricate balance of its two opposite forces — yin and yang.

Following numerous such observations, the Taoist philosophers came to name the two opposite forces **yin** (陰) and **yang** (陽). Yin, which literally means "dark" or "negative", is arbitrarily assigned to the softer, weaker and more passive of the two forces. In contrast, yang, which literally means "bright" or "positive", is arbitrarily assigned to the harsher, stronger and more active force. In our examples above, we have day time as yang and night time as yin; sun as yang and rain as yin; birth as yang and death as yin.

But what about the health of a human body? How does the philosophy of yin and yang apply to traditional Chinese medicine?

Sect. 1-6: The body's fuel tank as a bank account: vital substance and vital force

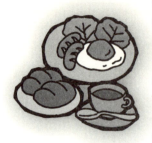

Vital substance is the energy you obtain from food.

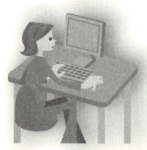

Vital force is the energy you spent for doing work.

Humans are a part of nature. Just like everything else in nature, the human body, according to traditional Chinese medicine, also operates on the basis of two opposite components — **vital substance** (水穀精微) and **vital force** (活力). Vital substance, the yin component, refers to the energy *input* acquired from the environment, which, at the most basic level, equates to food and water. On the other hand, vital force, the yang component, refers to the energy *output* used by the body for performing actual physical activities, such as running, seeing, listening, thinking, writing, talking, working and reproducing. This ancient concept, although derived from a philosophical origin, is fundamentally in agreement with the modern scientific definition of "living organism" — self-reproducing entities that are *capable of utilizing energy*.

Further extension of the theory of yin and yang would dictate that the wholeness, or health, of the human body depends on the proper balance of its two opposite components, vital substance and vital force — and it is very easy to understand why. First you must *acquire* energy (vital substance) from food, then you will be able to *generate* the energy (vital force) to perform work. Vital force, on the other hand, *consumes* vital substance and causes your body to go into a state of mini-crisis — hunger and fatigue — which stops your body from doing work and drives it to replenish its vital substance. In a healthy body, the two vital components alternately go up and down, as two children happily riding the opposite ends of a seesaw.

In this respect, the body is very similar to a machine, such as a car. However the body is much more complicated than that. With a car, you can keep driving until the fuel gauge drops to "empty", then you fill in more gasoline at a gas station and continue driving. With the body, unfortunately, you must be more cautious because this kind of practice is very dangerous.

You see, life in a modern society is very unpredictable. While a student, for example, may expect to work and study at a normal pace most of the time, there are the occasional quizzes, exams, projects and reports that require extra amount of energy and attention to handle — perhaps working for 16 consecutive hours or late into the evening as due dates approach. Needless to say, these occasional "emergencies" consume extra amount of vital substance. So, on any regular day, it is wise for him not to drain his vital substance completely empty but, instead, save up some of the energy each day in anticipation of those looming crises.

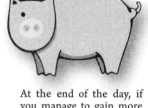

At the end of the day, if you manage to gain more energy than you spent, then you have some savings left in your bank account — that's vital essence.

In TCM, this extra savings for the rainy days is called **vital essence** (精). In banking terminology, we refer to it as "savings", or more appropriately, "long-term savings". All you need to do is to *deposit* more money into a bank account than you *withdraw* — by the end of the month, you will have made some "savings".

"Savings" is not the money you spend on everyday, expected necessities like clothing, food, rent and transportation (衣食住行); or regular bills like utilities and insurance. Rather, this is the money for once-in-a-long-time big-ticket items, such as a vacation to Hawaii, a big-screen plasma TV, fixing the car when it suddenly breaks down, patching the roof when it suddenly starts leaking, doctor's bill when someone in the family gets sick, replacing the old computer when it suddenly refuses to boot, a big wedding banquet when you get married and many other occasions that consume a lot of money but "have to be done" anyway.

> On any regular day, it is wise not to drain the vital substance completely empty but, instead, save up some in anticipation of looming crises.

What if a person does not have enough vital essence in reserve when a crisis occurs? Strange enough, the body does not immediately come to a halt but, instead, vital essence can be pulled from certain organs with less urgent need, such as the kidney and liver, to temporarily supply another organ in crisis, such as the brain. This practice of robbing Peter to pay Paul certainly relieves the immediate crisis, but if the situation prolongs or it occurs frequently, Peter will be very unhappy. That is why a person who regularly works overtime beyond his energy budget could find himself troubled by chronic diseases attributable to the depletion of kidney functions, such as tendinitis and lower back pain (according to TCM classification).

Certainly, building a strong reserve of vital essence is one of the most important strategies to maintain a healthy body.

Sect. 1-7: The body machine as a steam engine: chi

Thinking about the relationship between vital substance and vital force, you may realize that there has to be some kind of bridge between them. As vital substance is acquired from food, which is processed *locally* in the digestive tract, how is it possible that vital force materializes *globally* within the many organs throughout the body? According to TCM, that bridge in question is something called **chi** (or qi by mandarin phonics) (氣), a kind of energy in transit or an intermediate between vital substance and vital force. Chi streams along a series of interconnected channels called **meridians** (經絡) to supply energy to the many organs of the body. It is this energy flow that keeps the body alive.

The best way to illustrate this idea is to use the analogy of a steam engine. In a steam engine, water is boiled into steam by burning a fuel. The steam is then delivered, under high pressure, through pipes to the piston, which then generates motion when pushed by the steam.

In a locomotive, steam is pressurized and delivered through pipes to the steam engine. Similarly, in a human body, the chi is pushed and delivered through meridians to the organs.

Chi, which literally means "gas", can be thought of as the steam in a steam engine while the meridians which carry the constantly-moving chi can be thought of as the pipes that carry the steam. Furthermore, the chi has to be kept in a strong flowing current in order to continuously supply energy to the many organs — the same way that steam must be kept in high pressure if it is to reach the piston efficiently.

In fact, a whole system of therapy called **acupuncture** (針灸) has been established based on this concept of meridians and chi. TCM hypothesizes that when certain meridians become interrupted or blocked, the chi will not be able to flow smoothly and the organs fed by those meridians will subsequently be depleted of chi — leading to a decline of functions and, eventually, diseases. The solution is to stimulate the chi flow by inserting needles at specific points along the meridians called **acupoints** (穴位) which are accessible just underneath the skin surface. Once the chi flow resumes normally, health is restored.

The ancient art of acupuncture cures diseases by stimulating chi flow and clearing chi blockages within specific meridians.

Are these meridians real or imaginary? We do not yet know for sure. We do know that the meridians do not correspond to blood vessels, lymph vessels, nerves, muscles, tendons or other structures that are known to anatomists. However the acupoints along the meridians can be mapped by instruments that can detect the variations of electric field and electrical conductivity of the skin. So perhaps the meridians are not structural, but rather electromagnetic or biophysical, in a way that we have not yet thought of. Nonetheless, these acupoints have been tremendously useful for acupuncturists to treat diseases for millennia, which can be clinically verified by modern scientific methods.

Keep in mind that the theory of meridians and chi is a working hypothesis for traditional Chinese medicine and that it is being constantly modified and refined. Although we do not yet know its anatomical or biochemical basis, this fact should not diminish its value in medicine and science, as long as it has the power to account for observations and to predict experimental outcome — just like all other scientific theories. One only have to recall that when Gregor Mendel (1822-1884), the Austrian priest commonly known as "the father of genetics", discovered the laws of heredity through the experimentation with peas, DNA was totally unheard of — its role in carrying genetic information was not to be understood for another 80 years.

Certainly, one of the most important strategies in maintaining our health is to keep the chi flowing strongly and avoid any situations that can interrupt the meridians.

Sect. 1-8: The human body as a self-healing machine

We have been discussing the utilization of energy — the body's active or yang state — in the previous sections. Let us now shift gear to talk about another aspect of body functions — the resting state, regarded as the body's yin state. Although some people equate the resting state simply as an absence of activity or a loss of productivity, TCM tells us that this phase of life is just as important as the active phase in our daily rhythmic cycle — because this is the time when the body channels its vital essence inward to perform **self-healing** (自體癒合). You see, as we run our bodies at full speed during day time, we sustain and accumulate a host of wear and tear, damages, injuries and attacks on our bodies — our skin nicked, muscle fibers snapped, tendons sprained, neck and spine strained, nerves overexcited, bronchioles clogged by dust, arteries and veins stretched by blood, DNA damaged by ultraviolet light, tissues accumulate carbon dioxide and ammonia, and, above all, our systems invaded by environmental toxins, bacteria and viruses. All of these damages need to

> As we run our bodies at full speed during day time, we sustain a host of wear and tear, damages, injuries and attacks, which must be promptly repaired if our bodies are to operate actively for 80 years or more.

be promptly repaired if our bodies are to operate actively for 80 years or more — a lifespan which no car is known to achieve. Although our bodies try to deal with these "damages" immediately during the active state of the day, little energy is available to perform damage repair since most of our energy has to be channeled for physical activities like running, pushing, talking and thinking. It is not until we enter the resting state of the evening, commonly known as sleep, that the body's self-repair systems, which include the immune system, kick into high gear.

Just as you would turn off your washing machine before fixing it, you need to rest your body before it can be repaired.

Based on our daily experience, this actually makes perfect sense. When I caught a flu and was too incapacitated to go to work, I took a day off from work and — guess what I did at home? — slept through the day. I did not watch TV, even if I could, because I needed every bit of energy to be channeled to the immune system and to the healing process. When I caught a cold and came down with weeks-long lingering coughs, I could get rid of them only after several days of restful, plentiful sleep.

What happen if you habitually take inadequate rest? Most people can tell you that, during the day, they will have difficulties staying alert, have problems concentrating at work and may even fall asleep on the job. What is not so well recognized is that the body will not be able to finish repairing its damages by the time it needs to "take off" again in the morning — and serious problems will occur as non-repaired damages accumulate over time. Just imagine what will happen to an airplane that cannot complete its regular aircraft maintenance checks because it spends too little time on the ground — I don't even think I want to be riding that airplane.

That is why some of my patients suffer from shoulder and back pains that are very difficult to heal. Many of them, even those who considered themselves strong and muscular, could trace back to a particular instance of injury, like that time when she had to turn around a springbox to change the bed sheet — and sprained her shoulder. The patient was often amazed that such a seemingly light physical activity could cause such a painful injury. But what is even stranger is that such seemingly minor injury took months to recover, and, once recovered, re-injury could easily occur with another simple physical activity.

> Since these patients have been sleep-deprived, their ability to self-repair has been weakened for so long that many of the connective tissues have been deteriorating.

It turns out that most of these patients have been sleep-deprived, either due to long work hours or late-night entertainment. Their ability to self-repair has been weakened for so long that many of the connective tissues that support the shoulder and spine have been deteriorating — just not yet breaking. All it takes is a minor physical activity to cause heavy injury and, once injury occurs, the self-healing machinery is slow to carry out the necessary repair to return the tissues to normal.

Cancer is another good example that illustrates the importance of adequate rest. At the current state of science, many researchers recognize the existence of a link between stress and cancer as the rate of cancer has been observed to significantly increase among people who have experienced stressful or traumatic events, such as deaths of family members or divorces. Many researchers also suspect that the immune system plays a role in this phenomenon for it is a known fact that, during stressful time, the endocrine system, especially the adrenal cortex, produces stress hormones (e.g. cortisol) that prepare the body for a state of high alert while at the same time suppressing the immune system (which is why cortisol works as an immunosuppressant and anti-inflammatory drug). However, most researchers conclude that there is insufficient evidence that stress causes cancer and that stress probably only plays a very small role in cancer diseases.

I think it would be very helpful if we can look at the issues in a different perspective. Of course, it is not likely that stress will be proved to be a direct cause of cancer — because the direct causes of cancer are mutagens that cause DNA damages, such as environmental toxin, ultraviolet light and hepatitis B virus — while stress is apparently not a mutagen. But that will be missing the point. Perhaps the real question to ask is: if these common mutagens are often present in and around us, why aren't we *all* having cancer?

In fact, cancer cells occur spontaneously in our bodies in a daily basis — we just do not notice them because they are usually cleaned off by the immune system before they become noticeable. The immune system contains certain types of white blood cells, notably the cytotoxic T-cells and natural killer cells, which constantly patrol the body tissues and kill off abnormal cells, including cancer cells. This is why AIDS patients often suffer from Karposi's sarcoma, a rare type of cancer before the AIDS epidemic, since they do not have a functional immune system to clean up the cancer cells when they first appear.

> Stress causes deprivation of rest, which then leads to a depletion of immune functions. Under such circumstances, cancer cells escape our body's surveillance and multiply into full-blown tumors.

Stress does something similar — it causes deprivation of rest, which then leads to a depletion of immune functions as I have explained earlier. It is under such circumstances that cancer cells escape our body's surveillance and multiply into full-blown tumors. The stress or the lack of sufficient rest is only an indirect cause of cancer — but possibly a real cause nonetheless.

I have used three examples — flu, back pain and cancer — to illustrate how diseases occur as a result of a lack of proper rest. It should be clear that TCM views the yin activity of self-healing as part of a complete package of daily activities. That means if you perform yang activities, you must also perform yin activities — don't wait till you get an infection before allowing your immune system to work.

Certainly, one of the best strategies in maintaining our health is to ensure that our bodies receive plentiful rest and sleep so that they can effectively perform the innate self-healing process and maintain themselves in top condition.

Sect. 1-9: Once again, what is good health and what are good health habits?

We have taken a long journey through the many TCM concepts of body functions — vital substance, vital force, vital essence, chi, meridians, and self-healing. We are now ready to tackle the original question which we posted back in Sect. 1-4: what is the TCM interpretation of good health?

Just as an airplane needs regular aircraft maintenance checks to keep flying smoothly, just as a city street requires frequent paving and repairs to keep its surface in good condition, the key to a smooth running of the body is its ability to tap into its self-healing power to repair and revitalize its organs every day. Therefore, if the body is capable of efficiently carrying out this crucial process of self-regeneration, we are enjoying good health.

As we have explained, the self-regeneration process requires (1) plenty of vital essence in reserve, (2) strong chi flow to deliver the energy and (3) plenty of yin-state resting time. In order to ensure the high efficiency of self-regeneration, we must maintain a delicate balance of the yin and yang aspects of our bodies. Do you still remember what the yins and yangs are?

First of all, we have to maintain *a balance of the energy input from food (vital substance, the yin) and the energy output of physical activities (vital force, the yang)*. Not only do we have to have enough energy for external activities, we must also have enough energy to maintain a strong flow of chi and to afford a comfortable long-term reservation of energy (vital essence).

Secondly, we have to maintain *a balance of the active state (yang) and resting state (yin) of our bodies.* Since we tend to be overworked and over-stressed in this modern industrialized society, our main concern is usually the inability to obtain enough rest, particularly in the form of sleep. If we neglect to take our bodies back to the resting state, our self-healing process will not have the chance to complete its mission.

Ladies and gentlemen, this is why staying healthy can be so tricky, especially for those leading a high-flying life. We have to be mindful about how we are eating, working, exercising and resting every day in order to avoid disrupting the delicate balance of yins and yangs. The alternative, however, is much worse — our self-repair system will falter and diseases are the inevitable results.

So what are good health habits — the life habits that lead us to good health? The answer is now obvious: they are everyday practices that help us maintain the balance of yins and yangs of body functions, which then allows our self-regeneration system to keep us free from diseases. Do you know what these everyday practices are?

In fact, I have already mentioned them as we discussed the many TCM concepts in the previous sections (Sect. 1-6, 1-7 and 1-8). Here, I will briefly summarize them and save the details for the coming chapters:

First, we need to *maximize our acquisition of vital substance* by eating the right kinds of food and properly preparing the food for digestion (see Chapter 2 for more details).

Second, we need to *conserve our vital force* by carefully budgeting our energy expenditure according to the demands of our daily life (see Chapter 3 for more details).

Thirdly, we need to *strengthen our chi flow* by practicing special chi-enhancing exercises and therapies (see Chapter 4 for details).

Finally, we need to *be mindful about preparing our body for the resting state* just as we carefully plan and organize our daytime activities (see Chapter 5 for more details).

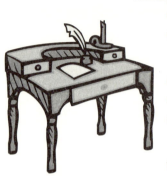

The four strategies to good health are like the four legs of a table — together, they can support an amazing amount of weight; but without any one of them, the table can easily topple over.

These four strategies are like the four legs of a table — together they keep your body that is the table top on solid ground. The good news is that there are no expensive pills to swallow, no surgery to perform and no costly products to purchase. However it does require that you take command of your free will and put the strategies into action. Remember: you are a human, not a car; and I am a physician, not a mechanic. You must be the central figure to take control of the destiny of your health — I, the physician, is only here to give advice.

And that is what I will do for the rest of the book.

CHAPTER 2
MAXIMIZING VITAL SUBSTANCE

Sect. 2-1: The downward spiral of poor digestion

Sect. 2-2: A tour of the digestive process: the beginning
        Goal of digestion. Oral cavity. Esophagus.

Sect. 2-3: Digestion in the stomach
        Stomach acid. Digestive enzyme. Stomach.

Sect. 2-4: Digestion and absorption in the small intestines
        Duodenum. Pancreas. Gall bladder. Small intestine. Liver.

Sect. 2-5: Elimination in the large intestine
        Large intestine. Resident bacteria. Fibers.

Sect. 2-6: TCM concept of digestion

Sect. 2-7: Eating well-balanced meals

Sect. 2-8: Eating fruit after lunch and dinner

Sect. 2-9: Accompanying each meal with a hot fluid

Sect. 2-10: Foods to avoid
    (a) *Cold foods and drinks*
    (b) *Raw foods*
    (c) *Direct-fire and deep-fried foods*
    (d) *Spicy foods*
    (e) *Overly sweetened foods*
    (g) *Supplements*
    (h) *Stimulants — caffeine, alcohol, cigarette and recreational drugs*

Sect. 2-11: Regular mealtimes

    (a) *Breakfast*

    (b) *Lunch*

    (c) *Dinner*

Sect. 2-12: Proper cooking methods

    (a) *Grains*

        White rice. Pasta.

    (b) *Vegetables*

        Water cooking. Stir-frying.

    (c) *Meat, poultry and fish*

        Steaming. Stir-frying.

Sect. 2-13: Practical tips for eating out

    Ice water. Hot drink before eating. Entree selection. Potlucks.

Sect. 2-1: The downward spiral of poor digestion

In the last chapter, we have discussed the importance of having a sizable reserve of vital essence for self-healing and for emergencies. Since VITAL ESSENCE = VITAL SUBSTANCE − VITAL FORCE (in other words, SAVINGS = DEPOSIT − WITHDRAWAL), one of the best ways to build our vital essence is to maximize the intake of vital substance. In this chapter, we will examine the many strategies we can use to do just that.

For most people, the process of acquiring energy (i.e. vital substance) from food is equivalent to the simple act of eating. True, there is a whole series of additional steps called digestion — but, since it is usually automatic and unnoticeable, most people just ignore it. So acquiring energy should be quite simple, right?

Well, there is actually more to the story. You see, digestion is an investment of energy, just as a business is an investment of money. In a business, you spend *money* up front to start a shop, then you make sales and you collect some money back — hoping to achieve a net gain called profit. That is the money you use to pay bills, buy things and, above all, continue running your business.

Needless to say, if business investment is that simple, we should all be wealthy businessmen by now. Why is that not the case? Well, because if you are not good at running a business, the profit you make can be so small that you have difficulties paying the rent and buying new inventory, just to keep your business afloat. Without the proper management skills, your business will constantly teeter on the verge of bankruptcy.

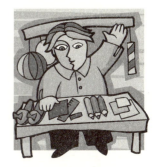

Food digestion is a business venture — whether you can make a profit from your investment depends on whether you have good management skills.

Digestion is just like business investment — you spend some energy up front to operate the myriad of organs of the digestive system, hoping that the *energy* released from the food will not only compensate for the energy you spent but also leave you a nice "profit" so that you can operate your brain, heart and legs. What many people do not realize is that if you are not good at running an efficient digestive process, you stand to make little or no gain in energy — and your *digestion business* itself will suffer, not just your brain, heart and legs.

Once this happens, the situation can quickly go from bad to worse. Now you can afford less energy to reinvest into your digestive system and, in turn, you will gain even less energy from food. The vicious cycle repeats — less energy gained leads to less energy invested, which leads to even less energy gained, which leads to even less energy invested, and so on. What starts out as a small hiccup in the digestive process can quickly spiral into a total dysfunction of the digestive system. This is what I call the "downward spiral of poor digestion".

Due to this unique nature, the digestive system is very prone to malfunction caused by minor disturbances. It is tantamount that we take very good care of the digestive system at all time, even when we are feeling upset or uninterested to eat. For this reason and the fact that it supports all organs of the body, TCM regards the digestive process as the most critical pillar in the maintenance of good health.

From my clinical experience, poor energy acquisition is one of the most common causes of many chronic diseases, including chronic fatigue, seepage of menstruation, restless leg syndrome (RLS), poor concentration and fibromyalgia, as most of the body functions in the patient are constantly running under starving condition. You will be surprised how many other "intractable" diseases are also caused by the inefficient procurement of energy.

Unfortunately, unlike business investments, we do not have the option of declaring bankruptcy in the business of digestion. The only option we do have is to learn to be a good energy investor.

> Poor energy acquisition is one of the most common causes of many chronic diseases, as most of the body functions are constantly running under starving condition.

Sect. 2-2:
A tour of the digestive process: the beginning

Why do some people have problems acquiring adequate energy? In the case of my patients, most of them were rather successful professionals who made a decent living — they had no trouble coming up with the money to buy food. But, consciously or unconsciously, they were not doing the right things to help the digestive process — and, with time, the downward spiral of poor digestion kicked in.

Now the real question is: how were they not helping the digestive process? In general, I can group the causes of poor digestion into three categories — (1) poor food choice (Sect. 2-7 to 2-10), (2) poor eating habits (Sect. 2-11) and (3) poor food preparation (Sect. 2-12). But to continue our discussion, it is necessary for us to first have a thorough understanding of the process of digestion so that we can later refer to some of its basic concepts.

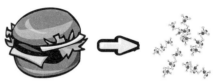

Digestion is truly a task of monumental proportion: a sandwich, for example, is so finely cut up that the resulting nutrient particles are only one-1,000,000,000th the size of the original sandwich.

Goal of Digestion. Digestion is the process of breaking down large chunks of food into tiny molecules of nutrients — so tiny that they can be absorbed through the inner lining of the small intestine into the capillaries. Thus, carbohydrates such as bread, rice, noodle and potato are broken down into simple sugar (glucose); proteins such as meat, fish, egg and milk are broken down into amino acids; lipids such as oil and fat (from meat, egg yolk and milk) are broken down into glycerol and fatty acids. Other nutrients, such as vitamins and minerals, are already small enough to be absorbed without further digestion, as long as they are released from the food matrix material, such as the cellulose cell wall of vegetable leaves.

Oral Cavity. Digestion begins in earnest as soon as food enters the mouth into the oral cavity. Here, the food is broken down mechanically by the chewing action of the teeth (#7, see the diagram of human digestive system), with the assistance of the tongue (#6) which strategically rolls and nudges the food in place. Note that we mammals are the only group of animals endowed with teeth designed for chewing so that we can release the energy from food as quickly as possible — a testament to our huge consumption of energy to support our high level of activities as well as to maintain a relatively high

Despite their fearsome appearance, the teeth of dinosaurs and other reptiles are useless for food digestion — they are only used for fighting and piercing. Only mammals, such as humans, have teeth capable of chewing.

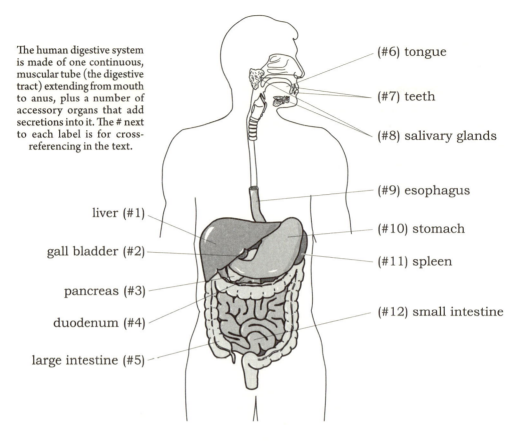

The human digestive system is made of one continuous, muscular tube (the digestive tract) extending from mouth to anus, plus a number of accessory organs that add secretions into it. The # next to each label is for cross-referencing in the text.

body temperature. (Reptiles do have teeth but they are used for fighting, hunting and piercing — they swallow their food whole.)

In the oral cavity, the very first station of the digestive system, digestion also occurs chemically — but only for starch. It is no wonder that almost all cultures eat certain varieties of starch-rich food as their main source of energy, be it rice, pasta, potato, bread, cereal, oat meal, cake or pie. The digestion of starch is achieved by a digestive enzyme called *salivary amylase* — which is secreted with *saliva* by the salivary glands (#8) and specializes in digesting *amylose*, another word for starch. You will encounter a number of digestive enzymes throughout the digestive tract — just think of them as tiny molecular scissors, each specializing on cutting up a certain food type (carbohydrates, proteins and lipids).

Esophagus (#9). After extensive chewing and mixing with saliva, the food chunks become slimy, minced boluses of crumbs. The boluses, lined up in single file, are then squeezed through a long fleshy tube called esophagus, just behind the windpipe, and into the stomach. This happens in a kind of slow motion, much like squeezing a tennis ball through a long, thick, narrow stocking.

Sect. 2-3: Digestion in the stomach

Stomach Acid. Once the food enters the stomach (#10), a ring-shaped muscle (cardiac sphincter) closes the junction between the esophagus and stomach so that the stomach content cannot reflux back into the esophagus. This makes sense because the stomach content is a sour, mushy paste mixed with hydrochloric acid, which is very corrosive and can injure the inner wall of the esophagus, giving it a painful, burning sensation. Incidentally, the occurrence of such burning sensation, called heart burn, is apparently quite common among adults (20% Americans have heart burn for at least once a week, according to WebMD!), which accounts for the numerous prime-time TV commercials selling over-the-counter quick-fixes for exactly this condition.

How does hydrochloric acid, the same chemical used in the steel industry to clean off rust, get in our stomach? Well, no, it doesn't come from our food; but our stomach wall contains numerous gastric glands which secrete hydrogen ions and chloride ions, which combine in the stomach to form hydrochloric acid. In order to contain the acid, a thin layer of mucus is produced to keep the acid from ever coming in contact with the stomach wall. This layer of protection is usually

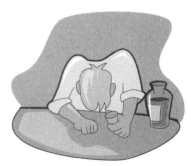

Besides giving you a convulsive hangover, alcohol can also give you stomach bleeding and ulcer.

quite effective but it is not foolproof, since the mucus can be dissolved away by certain chemicals like alcohol — which is why heavy drinking can lead to severe stomach bleeding.

So is the acid bad for us? No, the acid is present in the stomach for some good reasons. Normally it is very effective in killing microbes and parasites that enter the body with ingested food, thus keeping the intestines from being attacked by foreign invaders. One exception, however, is a bacteria called *Helicobacter pylori,* which can survive very well in the acidic stomach environment. Under certain circumstances (such as stress), the bacteria can undergo a sudden population explosion, causing massive infection and damages to the stomach wall — a condition commonly known as stomach ulcer. In addition, some viruses, such as Herpes, Hepatitis and Polio viruses, are capable of entering the bloodstream through the stomach wall before the acid can completely destroy them.

Digestive Enzymes. The hydrochloric acid also helps digestion by denaturing proteins and allowing pepsin, a protein-digesting enzyme produced by the gastric glands, to more easily attack the protein molecules. Imagine a normal protein molecule as a long ribbon that has been crumbled into a ball — just as protein molecules normally fold themselves into globules. Now imagine what happens when you throw this *ball* of ribbon up into the air — the ribbon unravels and unfolds into a relaxed piece of *string*, which is exactly what happens to protein molecules when they denature in acid. Once unfolded, the ribbon string can be cut up more easily with a pair of scissors than when it was still crumbled up.

Think of enzyme digesting food as a pair of scissors cutting a ribbon — the more relaxed the ribbon, the easier it is for the scissors to cut.

Finally, hydrochloric acid is needed to activate pepsin, the protein-digesting enzyme in the stomach. You see, the stomach itself is made of proteins too. So in order to avoid the stomach from being digested by its own digestive enzyme, pepsin is first secreted in an inactive form. When the boluses of food enter the stomach, the pressure felt by the stomach induces it to secrete hydrochloric acid, which then activates pepsin. Together with the fact that pepsin requires an acidic environment to perform its function, this arrangement makes sure that pepsin is active only when food is present for it to digest. But needless to say, if there is any disturbance to this delicate coordination of events, such as excessive secretion of acid during stressful time, pepsin may end up causing damage to the stomach wall.

Stomach (#10). Now let's shift our focus from the content inside the stomach to the stomach itself as an organ. The stomach is a muscular bag shaped rather like a miniature Scottish bagpipe. When it is empty, the stomach cavity collapses and the walls, wrinkled with folds, touch each other; when it is filled with food, the walls stretch and the cavity can expand up to a whopping 2 liters in volume — that's the volume of a party-size, 2-liter bottle of soft drink commonly sold in supermarkets. It surely holds a lot of food when packed to capacity — and that is exactly the main purpose of the stomach.

You see, while we usually take only a half to one hour to finish a meal, it takes three to four hours for all the food in the stomach to slowly empty into the very narrow small intestine (#12) — just as you pour oil slowly into a small-mouthed dispenser. Without a stomach, the food would have to drain directly from the esophagus into the small intestine — that would mean we have to spend four long hours at the dining table, three times a day. That is exactly what some people have to do after their stomachs are surgically removed due to stomach cancer — a very inconvenient life style indeed.

A human has a stomach for the same reason that a car has a fuel tank — it stores up a large amount of "food" to be slowly "processed" at a later time.

Incidentally, a surgical operation akin to removing the stomach, called gastric bypass, is becoming more and more common these days as a solution to the obesity epidemic. The surgeon staples off a large portion of the stomach, leaving only enough room to store a few mouthfuls of food. Then the food is rerouted directly into the small intestine, making it difficult for the patient to eat very much food but still feel satisfied with a "full" stomach.

This is indeed a very drastic operation and should only be considered for the extremely obese — keep in mind that the patient loses all the benefits of having a stomach and risks suffering from the many side effects associated with drastic weight loss. Unfortunately, the current trend appears to be that this operation is becoming more and more widespread. Considering how surgical procedures (e.g. plastic surgery) have been frequently sought after to solve problems from self-image to self-esteem, it is not very surprising that more people will seek gastric bypass as a quick and easy way to get slim. In any case, the surgery does nothing to address the underlying cause of obesity and unless the patient is able to remain on a strict diet for life, all the weight loss can disappear as rapidly as it was achieved.

As food enters the stomach, the smooth muscle of the stomach wall is stimulated to generate a wavelike, squeezing motion (called peristalsis) which churns the food and mixes it thoroughly with the gastric juice (acid, pepsin and water). By the time the food reaches the exit end of the stomach, the food has become a sterile, acidic, soft, consistent paste called chyme. It is now ready to enter, drip by drip, into the small intestine.

Sect. 2-4: Digestion and absorption in the small intestine

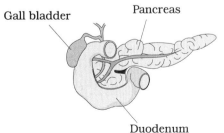

The duodenum receives pancreatic juice from the pancreas and bile from the gall bladder.

Duodenum (#4). The chyme, although partially digested, is still a long way from being fully digested into nutrients minute enough to be absorbed into the blood. It is no surprise, then, that the first part of the small intestine, the 10-inch-long, U-shaped duodenum, specializes in receiving more digestive juices from two accessory digestive organs — pancreas and gall bladder.

Pancreas (#3). The pancreas is probably well known as the organ associated with diabetes, since it is responsible for making the hormone insulin, which keeps our blood sugar level from soaring too high right after a meal. When the pancreas loses its function and fails to make insulin, the doctor prescribes the injection of recombinant insulin three times a day to avoid diabetic attacks. However, the pancreas also plays an important role in the process of digestion.

The pancreas is responsible for producing pancreatic juice — a sleuth of chemicals and enzymes capable of digesting all three major types of food (carbohydrates, proteins and lipids). The pancreatic juice also contains an alkaline salt called bicarbonate, which is used to neutralize the acidic chyme so that the digestive enzymes, which prefer a slightly alkaline environment, can work efficiently.

The neutralization of the acidic chyme is also necessary to protect the duodenum from being corroded. As you can probably imagine, any disturbance to the balance of the system, such as excessive production of stomach acid or faltering production of pancreatic bicarbonate or both, will tilt the pH towards the acidic side — leading to ulcer of the duodenum. In fact, 80% of all peptic ulcers (i.e. ulcers due to stomach acid) actually occur in the duodenum, not in the stomach — a testament to the delicate nature of the pH balance in the duodenum.

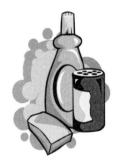

Bile released from gall bladder helps break down fat and oil in food the same way that detergent breaks up grease stains on dishes.

Gall Bladder (#2). Food containing lipids, however, presents an additional challenge. Since lipids do not mix well with water, the fats and oil tend to clump together into large blobs that are very difficult for digestive enzymes to attack. The solution is to apply a "detergent" called bile salt which is present in the bile released by gall bladder. Just like dish-washing detergent, bile salt has the ability to break up, or emulsify, large blobs of lipid into much smaller lipid droplets, thus allowing more surface area for digestive enzymes to work on.

The gallbladder, however, does not produce its own bile — it receives bile from the liver (#1). The main job of the gall bladder is to concentrate the bile and store the bile in large quantity for use during the next meal. Without the gall bladder, the duodenum still receives bile, but only in less concentrated form and in a slow, continuous trickle — whether or not food is present. That is why patients who have the gall bladder removed due to gallstones have to avoid ingesting too much fatty food in too short a time.

Small Intestine (#12). In the remaining 20 feet of the small intestine, the food is slowly moved forward by the squeezing motion of the small intestine while the digestive enzymes, those already mentioned and some additional ones secreted by the lining of the small intestine, are allowed time to continue their fine-cutting action on the food. As more nutrients are released from the food, they are absorbed through the lining of the small intestine and into blood vessels — and directly to the liver, the critical guardsman between the digestive system and the circulatory system.

Liver (#1). The liver, at 3 pounds, is the second largest organ in our body (behind the skin and equal to the brain) and is so versatile that medical textbooks identify over 500 different functions attributable to this one organ. We have already mentioned its role in producing bile for emulsification of lipids. An even more important role of the liver is to serve as a dam that holds the tide of in-coming nutrients from flooding the bloodstream of the body.

You see, one of the most difficult tasks of our body is to maintain a stable internal environment (homeostasis) for the cells while the external environment is constantly changing.

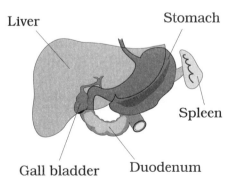

The liver is situated in the upper right abdomen, with the gall bladder tucked right underneath it. Just across the liver is the stomach, which occupies the upper left abdomen.

Take glucose (blood sugar), for example — a huge quantity rushes into the blood after every meal but our brain cells, among others, are very susceptible to such fluctuations. That is why, if the blood glucose level surges too high, a person will faint and lose consciousness — which indeed is the way many people first discover that they have diabetes.

So what can the liver do? When the flood of glucose enters the liver from the small intestine just after a meal, the liver, taking a cue from the insulin released by pancreas, has to quickly convert the glucose into glycogen (nicknamed "animal starch") and store it up as tiny granules within the liver cells — just as a potato plant stores up glucose in the potato spud in the form of starch. Later when the body consumes the glucose in blood and the glucose level begins to drop, the liver, taking a cue from a different pancreatic hormone called glucagon, converts the glycogen back into glucose and slowly release it back into the bloodstream. In this way, the liver can stabilize the glucose level in the bloodstream, regardless of what happens in the digestive tract.

Partly due to its strategic location as an interface between the digestive and circulatory systems, the liver also performs many functions related to the storage, synthesis and breaking down of many types of food-related biochemicals. It stores glucose (in the form of glycogen), minerals (especially iron) and many vitamins (including vitamins A, D, E and K). It synthesizes bile salt, glycogen, blood proteins (e.g. albumins, fibrinogens), cholesterol, phospholipids (for making cell membrane) and triglycerides (a common type of fat). It also breaks down excess amino acids, steroid hormones, aging red blood cells, toxins, drugs and alcohol.

The last item mentioned is the reason why heavy alcohol drinkers suffer from liver cirrhosis. Alcohol is toxic to cells — remember we use rubbing alcohol for sterilization — and the liver cells, as the first line of defense against food-borne toxins, fight valiantly to

Bile released from gall bladder helps break down fat and oil in food the same way that detergent breaks up grease stains on dishes.

break it down into less toxic acetaldehyde. But, if the alcohol enters the system in large quantity, the liver cells will die while performing its duty and will then be replaced by collagen fibers to fill their space (i.e. cirrhosis). Along with the loss of liver cells, the liver loses its functions — can you imagine? All 500+ of them, remember?

Sect. 2-5: Elimination in the large intestine

Large Intestine. By the time the digested food reaches the end of the small intestine, virtually all the absorbable nutrients and most of the water content have been absorbed through the lining of the small intestine. What is left is a thick slurry of indigestible waste and, still, plenty of water — something very similar to diarrhea. This material is moved into the 5-foot long large intestine to be prepared for elimination.

> The large intestine makes a final effort to retrieve as much of the water content as possible, the bulk of which originates from the gallons of lubrications and digestive juices secreted by the digestive organs themselves.

As animals living on dry land, we risks losing too much water and dying of dehydration. Therefore, the large intestine makes a final effort to retrieve as much of the water content as possible, the bulk of which originates from the gallons of lubrications and digestive juices produced by all parts of the digestive tract and its accessory organs. The large intestine also produces copious amount of mucus, which acts as a sticky glue to bind all the fecal materials into semisolid chunks for easier disposal.

Resident Bacteria. What materials make up the fecal waste? A significant part of it is bacteria that live inside the intestine, notably *Escherichia coli* or *E. coli* for short. When they are resident in the intestine, they are quite beneficial since they produce some vitamins B and vitamin K and prevent other types of virulent bacteria from living in our intestine. Use of antibiotics, therefore, may greatly reduce these resident bacteria, and, along with them, the many benefits they provide.

Fibers. Another type of indigestible waste is what we commonly called "fibers" — plant materials consisting mostly of cellulose. Cellulose is prevalent in all kinds of plant products since it is a carbohydrate that plants use to build their cell wall. Unfortunately, humans, unlike herbivores such as rabbits, horses and cows, lack the enzyme necessary for digesting cellulose. So much of the plant materials from vegetables and fruits simply pass through our digestive system undigested — and eliminated as waste.

So why should we bother to eat vegetables if we cannot digest them? Well, strange enough, precisely because they are not digestible. You see, the food moves along our digestive tract not because of gravity, but because of the non-stop wave-like squeezing motion (called peristalsis) of the digestive tract itself. How fast the intestine squeezes, however, depends on how much indigestible materials can be detected within its hollow space — the more fibers there is, the faster the intestine will squeeze.

Long, long time ago when our early ancestors were hunters and gatherers, the food they could find tend to be poor in calories and rich in fibers — which kept our ancestors' intestines very busy. Fast forward to the 21st century, with plenty of high-calorie and processed food easily available, the amount of fibers in our food has decreased so much that, quite often, our intestines cannot receive enough stimulation to maintain the proper rate of peristalsis, which means the waste stays in the small and large intestines for longer and a person may not feel the urge to go to the toilet for days. When he does finally go, the stool has become so dehydrated and hard that the experience becomes quite painful — a condition we call constipation.

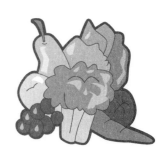

It was never a problem for our ancient ancestors who ate food with high fiber and low calorie. Today, however, we have to consciously remind ourselves to include plenty of vegetables in our meals in order to prevent constipation.

Prolonged constipation forces a person to exert prolonged and extra pressure on the bowel each time he goes to the toilet — and that is one of the most common causes of hemorrhoid, the swelling of the veins in the anus or rectum, which can cause extreme pain and, often, bleeding of the bowel. No wonder the most effective prevention for hemorrhoid is to soften the stool by changing to a diet with more vegetables and fruits.

There is another undesirable side effect with slow peristalsis — colon cancer. As the food content stays longer in our intestines, so do the environmental toxins, food-processing "ingredients" and agricultural chemicals that are ingested with the food. As a result, the intestinal lining greatly increases its exposure to these artificial and potentially carcinogenic substances, resulting in a greater chance of the intestinal cells to become irritated and form polyps — the precursors of colorectal carcinoma.

In any case, it is very important for us modern humans to consciously include a diet with plentiful roughage (i.e. indigestible plant materials) in order to keep our intestines active. Of course, we can also enjoy the bonus benefits of the unique minerals and vitamins present in vegetables and fruits. To use just one example: vitamin C, which is necessary for building the skin and blood vessels, can only be found in fresh vegetables and fruits, among all varieties of food.

Sect. 2-6: TCM concepts of digestion

As you will see, in spite of the fact that traditional Chinese medicine originated from a very different culture of a very different era than modern medicine, the TCM concepts of digestion align remarkably well with what we understand today through experimental science — allowing for some differences in the choice of technical terms.

For example, in TCM, the stomach is described as a "cooking pot" where the food is simmered by chi (recall the symbolic steam needed to drive a steam engine) and prepared into a form from which vital substance can be

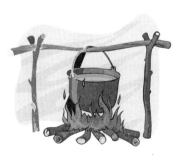

According to TCM, the stomach works as a cooking pot which simmers the food in order to extract the nutrients.

extracted. This is consistent with the fact that the food in the stomach is raised to our body temperature, adjusted to a specific pH and pulverized to a near-liquid texture in order to facilitate the action of digestive enzymes.

According to TCM, the function of the liver is to ensure the even and harmonious flow of blood and chi throughout the body by acting as a reservoir to hold back or to release blood into the bloodstream when needed. This description clearly corresponds to the role of the liver as a gateway between the digestive and circulatory systems, equalizing the levels of nutrients in the systemic bloodstream.

In TCM literature, the word "spleen" implicitly includes both the organs of spleen and pancreas, probably due to their close proximity. According to TCM, the "spleen" is a central digestive organ responsible for distributing vital substance throughout the body. It can be thought of as a distilling organ, similar to a spray bottle, which transforms food into a fine "mist" of vital substance, which is then "sprayed" outward through the network of meridians to all parts of the body. This idea corresponds very well with the role of the pancreas in producing the digestive enzymes necessary to transform food into microscopic nutrient molecules.

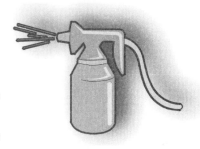

According to TCM, the pancreas ("spleen") works as a spray bottle which converts food into a mist, which is then distributed throughout the body.

The TCM implication of the "spleen" function is quite profound — the spleen must have strong spleen chi (recall our steam engine analogy in Sect. 1-7) in order to "pressurize" the chi within the meridians at all time. Therefore, if, for some reason, the spleen is weakened, the food cannot be transformed into the mobile, misty form and the immobile food materials will accumulate in the torso where they begin to "rot", causing a condition called "dampness" (濕重). As dampness becomes more severe, the spleen becomes overwhelmed, much like an overloaded pump trying to drain out flood water after a hurricane, and the network of meridians will become congested and clogged.

As we have discussed in Sect. 1-7, the blockage of chi flow in the meridians is one of the major causes of decline in organ functions and, ultimately, diseases. So how can we prevent this situation from occurring? By and large, the most common reason for the weakening of the spleen is poor food choice — which naturally leads us back to the topic of healthy habits for good digestion.

Sect. 2-7: Eating well-balanced meals

Now that we have a firm understanding of the process of digestion, we will dedicate the rest of this chapter on the discussion of health habits that promotes good digestion. To begin, I will take up the one question about eating that I am most often asked as a physician: what should I eat?

In our society, the notion of what a healthy diet constitutes has often revolved around the quest to lose weight and the fear of heart disease. In the last 40 years, we witnessed every possible type of nutrient scrutinized under the microscope and targeted to be the culprit of weight gain or heart disease — which, therefore, should be eliminated or reduced from our diet. The result? Depending on the popular fad of the year, the television and newspaper became saturated with advocacy (and commercials) for low-fat diet, low-carb diet, high-protein diet, low-calorie diet, low-trans-fat diet, low-saturated-fat diet, low-salt diet, high-fiber diet, low-cholesterol diet and, of course, no-meat or vegetarian diet.

> In our society, the notion of what a healthy diet constitutes has often revolved around the quest to lose weight and the fear of heart disease.

But how could protein, such as meat, be bad for one year and be encouraged to be the major food type for another year? How could carbohydrate be considered healthy for one year and the culprit of weight gain in another year? Can't the experts ever make up their mind? Is it healthy, anyway, to cut one type of nutrient drastically for the long-term in the name of health? Do we really have to micro-manage each and every type of nutrient just to eat healthily? Sometimes I wonder if the stress of worrying about the harm you may or may not get from eating, say, an egg actually causes more harm than benefit.

In TCM, instead of focusing on whether to raise or reduce a specific type of *nutrient*, we have a more holistic and user-friendly approach to healthy diet. Simply put, based on our understanding of the digestive system, TCM seeks the long-term balance of the three *major food types* — grains, vegetables and meats. As long as they are eaten in more-or-less the right proportion (see below), the liver, spleen and kidney will make the fine adjustment of distribution and storage according to the need of our body.

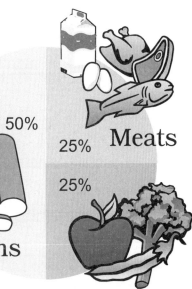

You don't have to be a nutrition scientist. In TCM, a well-balanced meal consists of apporoximately 50% grains, 25% meats and 25% vegetables.

Grains, such as rice, bread, noodle, oatmeal and potato, are rich in complex carbohydrates (mainly starch) which provide energy for both external and internal body activities. Obtaining energy is the main function of food, especially for those engaging in vigorous physical activities. Thus, grains, by itself, should make up the major part — about one-half — of our total diet.

Vegetables, including green leaves and stalks, orange carrots and tomatoes, provides the bulk of the roughage necessary to properly stimulate peristalsis of the intestines, as well as many unique vitamins and minerals not found in other types of food. Very often, people loathe or neglect to eat vegetable because it tastes bland and unpleasant — but it should not be so if properly cooked. That is why vegetables, which should make up about one-fourth of our total diet, should almost always be cooked before eaten (more on this in Sect. 2-10b).

Meats, as the name chosen for the last major food type, includes animal flesh and organs (including livestock, poultry, fish and seafood), egg and dairy products. These are foodstuffs that contain the animal protein necessary for building and repairing our body tissues and the fat necessary for building the skin, nerves (including the brain and spinal cord) and lipid hormones. Together, meats should make up the remaining one-fourth of our total diet.

Remember, the emphasis is on a balanced proportion of these three *food types* (grains, vegetables and meats), not the numerous kinds of *nutrient molecules* (simple sugar, complex carbohydrates, saturated fat, unsaturated fat, trans fat, cholesterol, essential amino acids, non-essential amino acids, fibers, iron, calcium, potassium, sodium, chloride, vitamins A, B, C, D, E, and on and on……). Whew! Isn't life so much easier?

Talking about meats, what about a vegetarian diet? Isn't that supposed to be more healthy? Unfortunately, there are many disadvantages of taking a diet devoid of animal proteins. True, certain plant-derived products, such as soy beans, are relatively rich in proteins — but only in comparison to other plants products. The bulk of plant tissues, mostly made of indigestible cellulose cell wall, is poor in protein since plants lack tissue mass that is built with protein, unlike muscles in animals. In order to obtain the same amount of proteins as you would from animal-derived food, you would have to ingest a huge amount of soy products — not an easy task if you rely on light versions of soy, such as soy-milk and tofu.

In addition, by chemical analysis, plant proteins are really not the same as animal proteins. Unlike animal

> Plant food alone does not carry the same animal chi that is necessary to support an active human lifestyle — work, play, laugh, think, talk, reproduce, etc.

proteins, proteins from any one type of plant tend to lack some of the ten essential amino acids required by humans — unless all ten are available, the proteins obtained are useless for human cells. Supposedly, this can be overcome by eating two different types of plants that are deficient in different types of amino acids — but that will mean one have to eat two times the original amount of plant materials in order to get a sufficient amount of the essential amino acids in question.

Along the same line, TCM considers animal proteins and plant proteins as unique and, therefore, not interchangeable. In fact, in TCM, every food item is considered unique with its own energetic and healing characters that affect a person differently — beef and pork are not the same, spinach and lettuce are not the same, even chicken breasts and chicken feet are not the same. For example, a patient with repetitive strain injury of the hands and wrists would be advised to eat animal parts with similar tendons, such as chicken feet or pig feet; a patient suffering from calcium loss of the bones would be prescribed broth made from pig bones; a patient with chronic cough would be required to drink broth made from pig lungs.

The extension of this concept is that since plants do not have animal features such as muscles, joints, tendons, blood, bones and brain, plant food alone does not carry the same animal chi that is necessary to support an active human lifestyle — work, play, laugh, think, talk, reproduce, etc. Therefore, the human body needs animal proteins to provide support to the body structures and activities specific to animals.

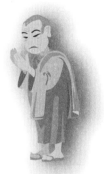

A vegetarian diet is only suitable for people with a sedentary lifestyle, such as Buddhist monks.

But you may wonder: aren't there people who do not eat meat? Yes, but, by and large, those who are successful doing so are people with specialized and sedentary lifestyles, such as Buddhist monks and nuns. People who lead an active lifestyle but forgo all animal proteins are prone to health problems related to protein deficiency, such as tendinitis, fibromyalgia, anemia, irregular or loss of menstrual cycles, impotency, osteoporosis and poor concentration. I have seen numerous patients in

> **HABIT #1:**
> Eat well-balanced meals with a mix of grains, vegetables and meats, roughly in the ratio of 50%-25%-25%.

such situations and, almost always, the fastest way to recover is to resume a normal intake of animal protein.

In summary, a healthy diet for a normal person should be well-balanced with a mix of grains, vegetables and meats, roughly in the proportions of 50%-25%-25%. You only need to focus on the kinds of food you put on the dinner table, not the exact number of grams and calories of each micro-nutrient on the labels. Your body will do the rest for you.

Regarding the summary statement above, let me make two quick remarks. First, notice that our major food types are grains, vegetables and meats — that means your dishes should be prepared and cooked from natural, unprocessed grains, vegetables and meats that are harvested from the source or purchased from the market. Most packaged foods are highly-processed or filled with artificial ingredients and, therefore, cannot be included in a well-balanced diet.

Second, the easiest way to ensure that the three food types are eaten in the right proportion is to simply take alternate bites of grain, and in between the grain, take turn to eat a bite of vegetable or a bite of meat. In my typical dinner, for example, I eat a bite of rice, then a bite of vegetable, then a bite of rice, then a bite of meat, then repeat the cycle (rice - vegetable - rice - meat). Whatever the size of your bite, the ratio of grain to vegetable to meat will come out to be roughly 2:1:1. Changing the flavor and texture in every bite also adds variations to the taste buds and is a good way to stimulate the appetite.

> **HABIT #2:**
> Prepare meals from natural, unprocessed grains, vegetables and meats, instead of packaged, highly-processed ingredients.

Sect. 2-8: Eating fruit after lunch and dinner

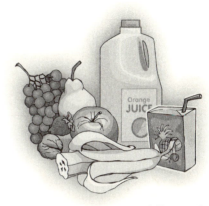

Fruits are a good source of fibers and vitamins, but should be avoided in the morning hours.

Fruits are good for their vitamins and as a source of fibers. They also stimulate the production of digestive enzymes. However, because fruits were designed for seed dispersal and are always eaten raw, they tend to have a purging and laxative effect on the intestines, which is undesirable when the digested food is still in the process of being absorbed. When the food moves too fast through a hyperactive intestine, there will not be enough time to fully absorb the water and nutrients, resulting in loose stool and frequent visits to the toilet.

Therefore, one should avoid eating fruit in the morning (from 5 A.M. to 11 A.M.), a time when the key digestive organs are most active absorbing the final nutrients from the meals of the previous day. Over-stimulating the digestive tract at this time will cause a drainage of nutrient despite the huge amount of energy invested in the digestion of the food. This applies to fruit of all forms, including fruit juice, slices over cereal, dried fruit and whole fruits.

The best time to eat fruit is right after lunch and dinner. Moderate amount of fresh fruit eaten at this time can enhance the secretion of digestive enzymes from the digestive tract and the accessory organs. But because the fruit is cushioned with a relatively large amount of other food that has already entered the stomach, its purging effect is reduced to a minimum.

In any case, even though fruits are considered to be good for our health, they should be eaten in moderate amount in order to avoid their purging effect and possibly throwing off the balance of the major food types.

HABIT #3:
Eat a moderate amount of fruits after lunch and dinner to stimulate digestion, but avoid them in the morning.

Sect. 2-9: Accompanying each meal with a hot fluid

Most people have experienced the discomfort of indigestion after gulping down a few bites of dry, cold (not warmed) meat or biscuit. The cause of the indigestion has to do with the biochemistry of digestive enzymes — they only work efficiently if the food is first thoroughly mixed with water and raised to the body temperature of 99°F (37°C). When the food is cold and dry, it takes an unusually long time to get thoroughly wet and warmed, causing your stomach to experience distress in the form of indigestion.

With this knowledge in mind, we can easily understand the many benefits of preceding a meal with a hot fluid, such as a hot broth or a nutritious drink. Remember that TCM considers the stomach as an oven that simmers the food in preparation for digestion? Drinking half to one cup of hot fluid before a meal can effectively lubricate our esophagus and pre-heat the oven that is our stomach. Drinking another half to one cup of hot fluid after meal also serves to cleanse and further moisten the digestive tract.

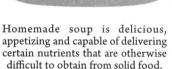

Homemade soup is delicious, appetizing and capable of delivering certain nutrients that are otherwise difficult to obtain from solid food.

Hot fluid also has a bonus benefit that is not well recognized — the ability to provide nutrients in a soluble form that is easy to absorb. For certain types of nutrients, the liquid form may be the *only* form that can be efficiently absorbed. A good example is calcium, which many people try to supplement by taking *solid* calcium pills in the form of calcium carbonate (i.e. pure chalk which teachers use to write on blackboards), which is totally insoluble in water. The calcium pills can only be dissolved by reacting with the acid in stomach but this reaction consumes stomach acid, may upset the natural pH of the stomach, takes a long time and still does not dissolve to completion. At the end, the amount of soluble calcium available is very low.

In contrast, a soup made from pig bone or fish bone has none of the drawbacks of the synthetic supplements. When pig bone is boiled in broth for two hours, the natural matrix-bound calcium, such as calcium chondroitin sulfate, is extracted in soluble, liquid form. This is the kind of calcium that can be readily absorbed and used for the building of bones. Incidentally, many food supplement companies have jumped on the bandwagon of selling *pills* of chondroitin sulfate (sometimes marketed as "glucosamine") — but why pay big dollars for *pills* if we can get it cheaply from a soup?

Needless to say, homemade broth or soup is the best choice for pre-meal and post-meal hot drink. Unlike in American cuisine, where the soup is often considered an optional side dish, a hot soup is the essential anchor of a meal in Chinese cuisine and is always served before the main dish. In Hong Kong, even fast food restaurants include a hot broth with the meal package, and in many Chinese restaurants in San Francisco, you can request the soup of the day for free with a purchased meal. At home, it is customary for Chinese families to prepare hot broth with specific combinations of herbs and meat according to the climate to effect natural healing and to boost immunity — a practice commonly known as food therapy (食療).

> **HABIT #4:**
> Drink a hot fluid, such as soup, seed-based nutritious drink, herbal tea or hot water before and after a meal to pre-heat and lubricate the digestive tract.

However, if broth or soup is not available, the next best choice is a hot seed-based nutritious drinks. These drinks can be made from the original ingredients in your own kitchen or, when time is in short supply, purchased from most Oriental grocery stores in convenient powder form. Examples of seed-based drinks are almond drink, black sesame seed drink, peanut drink, walnut drink, water chestnut drink, Ovaltine (a malted drink), rice milk and soy milk. They are delicious without additional sweeteners and serve well as pre-meal hot drink to pre-lubricate and pre-warm.

If you are in a restaurant where neither broth nor seed-based nutritious drink is available, go for hot non-caffeinated herbal tea (always served in Chinese restaurants), warm dilute fruit concentrate (e.g. black currant) or even hot water for the pre-meal warmth and post-meal cleansing. Nothing is worse than starting a meal cold and dry.

Sect. 2-10: Foods to avoid

Just as we need to know what food to eat to maintain our health, it is equally important that we know what food to avoid. It may come as a surprise to some people, but many of the foods that should be avoided are commonplace in American culture and are consumed without much thought with regard to our health. It could be difficult for a person to change a habit that he has been practicing since childhood, but when you reach mid-age of your life or when your body is feeling not as durable as before, consider my explanations below, experiment on amending your eating habits accordingly and look for signs that your body is benefiting from the changes you make.

(a) Cold drinks and foods

Sit down at a restaurant table and I will be greeted by a smiling (hopefully) waiter bearing a tray with tall glasses of ice water — water so chilly that, just one sip later, my teeth feel numbed and loosened from the gum. What a great way to start a dinner!

But seriously, icy cold drinks like ice water, iced tea, iced coffee, cold soda, chilled fruit juice, cold punch, etc. are not good ways to prepare the digestive system for a meal. These drinks stun the digestive tract, slow down peristalsis, inhibit the flow of digestive

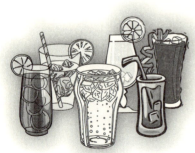

Iced water, iced soda, iced punch and iced cocktail chill the stomach, disrupt peristalsis and inhibit digestive enzymes — definitely the wrong way to start a meal.

juices, cause blood vessels to constrict and hinder absorption. When chilled by the cold, the stomach has to first spend chi to raise its own temperature, as well as the temperature of its content — from 0°C of the ice back to 37°C of the body. As a result, a huge amount of energy is wasted and the process of digestion is delayed — greatly reducing our "profit" in our business of "energy investment".

> **HABIT #5:**
> Avoid cold drinks and cold foods during regular meals; instead, heat them up or replace them with hot alternatives.

Then what should we drink? Of course, a hot fluid — broth, soup, seed-based drink, tea or water, as we have already discussed in Sect. 2-9. In any case, nothing icy cold, please.

Sometimes I suspect that the practice of cold drink might have been derived from the convenience of refrigeration to preserve food, as evidenced by the fact that even toddlers are taught to fetch and drink from their milk bottle directly from the refrigerator. Unfortunately, this causes a whole range of health problems, including stomach upset, indigestion, curd regurgitation and intestinal gas, in many of my baby patients — due to the simple fact that the young digestive tract is very irritable by cold temperature. True, as the practice of drinking cold milk becomes a habit, many babies develop a tolerance against cold but it is hardly a healthy practice, especially when they are otherwise weakened. The simple solution: take a little time to warm up the milk before drinking.

Many types of dessert has to be served cold, however, such as ice cream, frozen yogurt, jelly, pudding, popsicle, yogurt, etc. These are fine as desserts to be eaten for fun (not for nutrition) in small amount in a warm summer day — but not as the main part of a meal and, definitely, not in a cold winter day. Do not skip meal to eat ice cream — it is fun to eat, but not easy for digestion.

> **HABIT #6:**
> Eat small amount of cold dessert occasionally for fun and only in a warm day.

(b) Raw foods

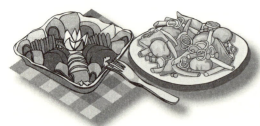

Plant materials, when eaten raw, are tough for the digestive system while much of the vitamins and minerals remain inaccessible inside the cellulose cell wall.

The green salad, another American staple, is considered by some to be one of the healthiest items on the menu. What can go wrong with a plate of freshly washed and chopped lettuce leaves, spinach leaves, cucumber slices, carrot slices and peas? Well enough, except for one problem — it is almost always served raw, making it very tough, both literally and figuratively, for the digestive system to handle.

Some people reason that vegetable should be served uncooked because the heat and water from cooking can destroy or wash away the vitamins and minerals. There is some truth to this thought but one has to understand that the vitamins and minerals are present in the juice, which is locked up within the box-like cell wall compartments of the leaves. However, as we have discussed in Sect. 2-5, the cellulose cell wall is indigestible by humans except for some minimal mechanical chewing. This leaves most of the juice trapped and unharnessed within the cell wall compartments, only to be expelled as waste at the end.

Cooked vegetable, on the other hand, offers two advantages over uncooked vegetable. First, the heat of cooking physically breaks open the cellulose cell wall of plant tissue, releasing the juice and making it available for absorption. You can observe this process by placing a piece of lettuce leaf in boiling water and notice how, within 30 seconds, the rigid sheet collapses into a small, soft crumb — the huge decrease in volume is due to the breakdown of the cellulose cell wall and the collapse of the cell wall compartments. True, a portion of the vitamins is destroyed but, when cooked briefly, the huge amount of additional vitamins unlocked from the cell wall more than make up for the loss.

> HABIT #7:
> Always cook vegetables before eating to soften the plant tissue and to release the vitamins from the cell wall.

The second advantage of cooking should also be obvious — the cooked plant material is much softer and much smaller to eat. Do an experiment by cooking your regular bowl of green salad, either by stir-frying or boiling in water, and you will find that a large bowl of tough green is equivalent to only a few mouthfuls of soft, cooked leaves. It is easy to eat three to four times as much vegetables when they are cooked — how about that for more vitamins and minerals?

I do have a few American friends who hate cooked vegetables because it tastes bad — citing the all-too-common "green pudding" (i.e. boiled broccoli) that was force-fed to them during childhood. That was obviously an unfortunate case of overcooking — which not only makes vegetable unpalatable, but also causes unnecessary loss of nutrient. It is, therefore, very important to learn the proper cooking techniques to both enhance the taste and preserve the nutrition (more in Sect. 2-12).

Learn proper cooking methods to enhance the flavor of vegetables. Poor cooking techniques, however, can make vegetables unpalatable.

(c) Direct-fire and deep-fried foods

In any occasion of festivity or celebration, we can expect someone to roll out a grill for BBQ — grilled hamburgers, charbroiled steaks, barbecued ribs, chicken legs and turkey legs. Even corncobs, cucumbers, carrots and marshmallows can be roasted on the grill. If not, there will surely be plenty of deep-fried party foods, such as fried

A sample of barbecued, roasted and deep-fried foods — mostly food for special festivities. They are crunchy and fun for parties but too dehydrated for the digestive system if eaten regularly in everyday meals.

chicken wings, crispy French fries, crunchy fried potato or corn chips, fried chicken nuggets and fried fish fillet.

Such foods cooked with direct fire or high heat are fun to the taste buds but are actually very taxing to the digestive system. The intense heat during grilling or frying drives off much of the internal moisture from the food. Due to their dry texture, once inside the digestive system, the foods will withdraw a large quantity of moisture from your body — costing extra expenditure of vital substance for digestion and leaving your body in a state of dehydration (熱氣).

> HABIT #8:
> Avoid eating direct-fire and deep-fried foods in regular meals.

In addition, while the charring of BBQ creates plenty of indigestible carbon particles, the oil used in deep-frying introduces large quantity of fat into the food — both require extra time and energy for the digestive system to handle.

True, we still have to face reality — for as long as there are festivals and celebrations, direct-fire and deep-fried foods are probably an inescapable part of social life. But, keep in mind, they are meant for special occasions only. Most importantly, you should consciously avoid direct-fire and deep-fried foods in your regular daily meals — save the chance for a special occasion.

(d) Spicy foods

Isn't it hilarious how some American fast food restaurants try to lure customers by boasting their offering of spicy foods on TV commercials? One TV commercial showed two tough-looking men in a salon, dressed in cowboy attire and in the stance of a gunfight, but were actually competing to see who can better tolerate the new, extra spicy sandwich sold by this fast food restaurant.

Hot sauce and chili pepper are infamous for making people breathe fire out of their mouths.

Needless to say, the loser was the one who ended up running outside just in time to dunk his fiery, smoking head into a trough of cold water. Is that really the kind of experience that customers look for when they patronize a fast food restaurant?

Oh, yes, I know that was supposed to be funny — just a joke, right? But spicy foods laced with red hot salsa, sinus-cleansing horseradish, tongue-biting curry, fire-alarm chili and hot sauces containing black pepper, cinnamon, mustard or chili pepper do indeed jolt a person simultaneously with a stinging sensation and a numbing sensation. Although seasoned consumers will develop tolerance against such jolts and even begin to interpret them as pleasurable tingles on the tongue and mouth, I can assure you that there is nothing pleasurable for the internal organs, especially the stomach, heart, liver and kidneys.

Why the heart? When the body is under attack by stimulating, spicy food, its immediate response is to adopt a fighting mode in defense — the overall metabolic rate increases, the heart beat rate rockets, the body temperature is raised, profuse sweating ensues, and blood is diverted away from the digestive system. When you are already hungry and tired, the last thing your heart needs is to race as if an imaginary bear is in hot pursuit.

Why the liver and kidneys? Much of the burning sensation of spices is due to a chemical called capsaicin (the same active chemical used in the crowd-control device pepper spray), which is a neurotoxin that over-stimulates nerve cells, much the same way MSG (monosodium glutamate, a seasoning chemical) causes headache in some people. Naturally, while the liver kicks into high gear to have the spicy neurotoxin detoxified, the kidneys also try to purge it by washing it out of blood and into urine with water. Not only do these extra works exhaust the liver and kidney, but they also count towards the expenditure column of our energy budget.

> HABIT #9:
> Stay away from spicy foods to prevent exposing your internal organs from overstimulation.

As a final note, the burning sensation of capsaicin is generated through a neural pathway specific for pain — typically used as a warning signal for chemical and physical dangers. Don't you think the body is trying to tell us something about spicy foods?

(e) Garlic

In my opinion, garlic is a much misunderstood item. A lot of health food outlets promote garlic as a healthy food, stating that it kills bacteria, reduces formation of blood clots and boosts the immune system. They even state that the Chinese people, in all their wisdom, use garlic in their cooking.

True, you'll find garlic used quite often in Chinese cooking, especially in restaurant dishes. But the garlic, usually crushed or minced, is only used as a flavoring agent when stir-fried along meat and vegetable. It is never meant to go into one's mouth and definitely not one's stomach!

In Chinese cuisine, garlic is only used as a condiment and is never intended to be eaten.

In TCM, garlic is considered a powerful stimulant and is used to treat specific diseases. However, for cooking (not eating) purpose, it can often be over-stimulating when more than one or two cloves are used. It is definitely unsuitable for ingesting in any significant amount, especially when raw or roasted.

What happens when one does ingest garlic? By its nature, garlic strongly draws moisture from internal organs, causing dryness of the throat, lungs and mucus membranes in general. Its stimulatory effect often manifests in the form of insomnia — particularly evident in people who are already over-stimulated by late-night work or late-night entertainment.

> **HABIT #10:**
> *Avoid the use of garlic in cooking and never ingest garlic to prevent over-stimulating the body.*

People who are hyperactive, whether physically or mentally, should avoid food containing garlic and even dishes cooked with garlic.

(f) Overly sweetened foods

Partly due to the low cost of high-fructose corn syrup, the supermarket is awash with overly sweetened, highly-processed, packaged foods. You cannot avoid passing by them every time you have to walk all the way to the back to fetch milk or meat — ice cream, candies, chocolate, frosted cakes, cookies, frosted cereals, flavored chips, soda drinks, fruit juices and jelly donuts, etc. Even foods that are not supposed to be sweet contains sweetener as flavoring — ketchup, mayonnaise, sauces, porridge, oat meal and cereal bars, etc. They are everywhere!

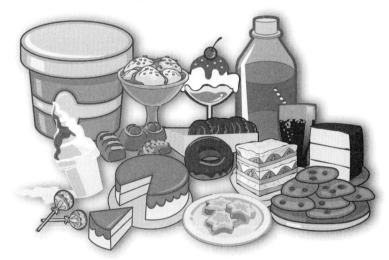

Humans are genetically programmed to crave sweet food as a way of survival. But when highly sweetened foods become so easily available in modern society, our instinct is causing us to overload ourselves with sugar.

Most packaged foods are produced in the factory with highly-refined ingredients by highly-processed methods. In the quest for artificial cosmetic appeal, prolonged shelf life, more attractive taste, lower manufacturing cost and higher profit margin, the food companies take apart and alter the original ingredients, put them together with heavy foreign flavoring and chemical preservatives, and package the products in colorful wrappings — resulting in the loss of nutrition and flavor of the original ingredients. So what is the purpose of food, again? Not to worry, they say, many products have been fortified with extra vitamins and minerals — breakfast cereal and fruit drinks come to mind. Are these really necessary?

The main problem with large dose of simple sugar is that it is rapidly absorbed without much digestion. This sudden flooding of the bloodstream with sugar causes a huge burden on the pancreas and liver, which have to decrease the blood sugar level in an equally rapid rate (see Sect. 2-4, Liver). Much of the glucose has to be stored in the liver and any excess glucose has to be converted into fat and stored under the skin — the beginning of obesity.

> As the pancreas and liver are repeatedly overwhelmed with exhaustive workloads, the liver slowly becomes desensitized to insulin and eventually stop responding to insulin altogether.

As the pancreas and liver are repeatedly overwhelmed with exhaustive workloads, the liver slowly becomes desensitized to insulin due to chronic exposure to elevated level of insulin. Eventually the liver will stop responding to insulin altogether (a condition known as insulin resistance), failing to store up glucose and releasing large quantity of glucose into the systemic bloodstream. The blood sugar level becomes so abnormally high that the kidney has to release much of it in urine — the beginning of type II diabetes mellitus. Not surprisingly, the abundance of overly sweetened foods is suspected to be the cause of recent increase in type II diabetes in young people.

It should be clear now that overly sweetened foods is a heavy burden to the liver, pancreas and kidney. Many food companies come up with diet versions of the same foods — but the artificial sweeteners used to substitute sugar is just as harmful because they are regarded as unnatural toxins that need to be detoxified and eliminated by the liver and kidney. The best way to avoid them is to stay away from packaged foods and to stick with foods cooked

> HABIT #11:
> Avoid eating overly sweetened, packaged foods to prevent from overworking the pancreas, liver and kidney.

from original fresh materials, usually found at the back and periphery of the supermarket.

Notice that the issue here is not whether to eat sugar, but how much sugar to eat. While we should avoid overly sweetened foods, moderately sweet foods should be appropriately incorporated into our daily diet to provide variety to the menu. There is nothing wrong with using a small amount of sugar as a sweetener in a warm glass of cow milk or soy milk, in seed-based drink, in meat marinade sauce and in light dessert.

The trouble is: some people, when in a hurry or a bad mood, skip the regular meal and replace it with three pieces of ultra-sweet chocolate bars. This is very damaging to their health.

(g) Supplements

Vitamins, minerals, fatty acids and amino acids are good for us. Therefore, a lot of people think, more of them must be better. Capitalizing on such skewed psychology, the dietary supplement industry has produced a bewildering myriad of pills to satisfy everyone who believe an extra boost of nutrients is necessary to stay healthy.

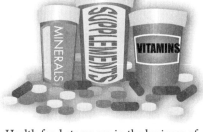

Health food stores are in the business of selling pills of concentrated minerals, vitamins and other dietary supplements. But do they make you more healthy?

To be sure, if one is eating a well-balanced diet, one should already have acquired enough nutrients of any kind from food alone. If one is concerned about lacking a certain type of nutrient, the best solution is to acquire more from its natural sources — liver for iron, bone soup for calcium, fruit for vitamin C, a walk in the morning sun for vitamin D. Nutrients obtained from natural sources are cheaper, more readily utilized by the body, free of artificial additives and have the bonus benefit of focusing your attention on eating for good health.

Supplements in pill form are nothing more than concentrated nutrients that rapidly flood the system and are then just as rapidly eliminated by the liver and kidney — just like anything that is in huge excess at any one time. Even worse, if the system cannot get rid of the excess nutrients, they clog up the meridians like a traffic jam, creating a huge burden on the spleen which finds it difficult to "pump" vital substance through the clogged meridians. By ingesting supplements, you managed to increase the workload for the liver, kidney and spleen, making your energy investment less profitable — not to mention the money invested on the supplements themselves.

> HABIT #12:
> Avoid taking supplements as a source of nutrients — instead, obtain nutrients from natural sources.

Supplements are seldom beneficial except when a person is critically and acutely lacking certain nutrients due to serious disease condition. For the long term, a well balanced diet is the only way to ensure adequate nutrients.

(h) Stimulants — caffeine, alcohol, cigarette and recreational drugs

Stimulants are used by many people to alter their moods by directly interfering with the normal functions of the brain. Caffeine, commonly delivered in the form of coffee, is used by tired and sleepy people to stay awake. Alcohol is used by unhappy people to feel unworried. Cigarette is used by anxious and stressful

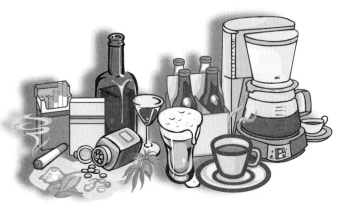

Some people feel the need to constantly supply themselves with mood-modifying chemicals or else their lives become either too dull or too stressful to enjoy. Not surprisingly, the international trade of these psychedelic chemicals make up a huge part of the global economy.

people to feel relaxed and in control. Recreational drugs, such as cocaine, marijuana, amphetamines and psychedelics etc., are used by depressed people to experience a moment of euphoria.

The harmful effects of these stimulants are well-publicized in the media and are familiar even to the users of the stimulants themselves. The most directly affected organ, of course, is the brain because it is forced by the biochemical effects of the drugs to function in a way that it is least capable of functioning — to be awake when tired, to be unworried when unhappy, to be relaxed when anxious, to be euphoric when depressed. The result is that the brain finds itself totally exhausted and disoriented once the effect of the drug disappears — heavy coffee drinkers quiver uncontrollably without their morning coffee; alcohol drinkers experience the notorious hangover the next morning; cocaine users often sleep for three consecutive days after an episode of euphoria, totally oblivious of thirst and hunger.

Besides the nervous system, all chemical stimulants set off serious, chronic side effects on the rest of the body. For example, caffeine is a diuretic, which causes frequent urination and rapid loss of water (dehydration) and minerals (chemical imbalance). Alcohol causes the loss of liver cells as they die in an effort to detoxify the alcohol (liver cirrhosis) — and the loss of many of the 500+ vital liver functions we discussed (Sect. 2-4 and 5-3) (this also applies to long-term use of any drug). Smoking causes lung cancer, chronic bronchitis, emphysema, coronary heart disease and atherosclerosis (blockage of blood vessels).

As for recreational drugs, the Chinese equivalent for the term is "poisonous substance" (毒品), which makes it clear that using drug is equivalent to poisoning the body while everybody understands, with no ambiguity, that the eventual outcome of taking a "poison" is death. It is notable that Chinese language does not suffer from a semantic

> The use of stimulants often begins as a way to self-medicate symptoms of fatigue, depression, anxiety, stress and despair — often the byproducts of poor health habits in the first place.

ambiguity similar to that of the English word "drug", which often muddles the boundary between "drugs that heal" and "drugs that kill". Conversely, the English term "recreational drug use" downplays the danger of drugs by muddling "suicide by poisoning" with the idea of "having fun with funny chemicals".

One may ask: if these psychoactive stimulants are well-known for their long-term health hazards, why are so many people still using them? Most of these people are motivated by the desire to and promise of feeling better physically and emotionally. The use of stimulants often begins as a way to self-medicate symptoms of fatigue, depression, anxiety, stress and despair — often the by-products of poor health habits in the first place. Unfortunately, although the stimulants initially produce quick relief, the fact remains that the cause of the symptoms have not been addressed. As a result, the symptoms persist as soon as the stimulant dissipates, and soon, the users have to reach out for the drugs again for another chance of quick relief. Once this becomes a habit, the users become dependent on the drugs just to sustain normal body functions and the drug habit becomes very difficult to stop.

> HABIT #13:
> Eliminate the need to use stimulants by identifying and correcting the faulty living habits that are causing your health problems.

So what is the solution? Since the root of the symptoms lie in poor health habits, the only way to return the body to good health is to identify the problems and transition into healthy living habits that correct the problems. Some people refuse to do so because this method takes time and requires persistence to succeed — it will last much longer and cost much less to accomplish. Don't be fooled by promises of quick fixes!

Sect. 2-11: Regular mealtimes

Now that we have finished the discussion on what to eat and what not to eat, we will change our focus on the proper ways of eating.

The first important rule to remember is that we should eat three well-balanced meals every day at regular, predictable times — breakfast, lunch and dinner. For many people, this can easily be accomplished within the rigid schedule of a school day or work day — you have to finish breakfast before leaving home by a certain time, your work place may already have a designated lunch hour and you leave your office at a fixed time, commute, cook and eat dinner at home.

But I am sure you know of friends or coworkers who have a completely different idea about mealtimes. To be sure, in the life of a busy person, there are plenty of unforeseen events and needs that tend to put basic activities like eating in a lower priority. Consider a typical day of the following fictional white-collar worker, a composite of several of my patients:

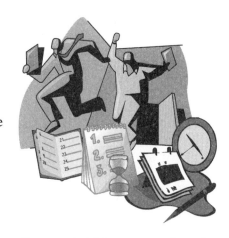

Since he went to bed late the previous night, he is barely half-conscious by the time he has to leave home. No time for breakfast — so he quickly take a cold shower on the head to wake himself and leave for work. Instead of feeding the body with nutritious food, he grabs a cup of dark, smelly, wake-up coffee on the way and, appearing fresh and alert, he steps into the office.

When a person's life turns into a chase after the clock, as dictated by his appointment book and to-do list, it is very easy for him to overlook mundane and less important routines such as eating and sleeping.

Too busy to worry about hunger, he attends meetings and works on the computer with as much energy as he can muster. Half past noon, his colleagues go out for lunch but he needs some extra time to finish a report due at 5 P.M. So he grabs a bag of BBQ-flavored potato chips and a banana, eats while continues on with work.

In the afternoon, coworkers in the office are passing around packaged snacks — candies, donuts, gummy licorice, dried fruits, roasted nuts, popcorn and more chips. He grabs a handful whenever his hands are free, staving off the hunger caused by his skimpy lunch.

Finally, it's 5 P.M. Whew, what a close call — but at least the report went in before the deadline. He does not feel very hungry after all that snacks but the day-long stress needs to be soothed. So he went with a few coworkers to a nearby pub, just in time for the discounted happy hours. A few glasses of beer and plenty of gossips later, life seems to be more relaxing — or is he just numbed? Time to go home.....

It is almost 9 P.M. and he realizes he hasn't eaten anything seriously the whole day. What to eat for dinner? Well, too tired to cook, he decided to pick up a grilled-beef hamburger, some French fries and an ice-cold soda on the way home. The fast-food dinner, while heavily flavored, feels more like a bulging lump in the stomach that refuses to disappear.

It is 11 P.M. and the thought of going to bed crosses his mind — but what about that DVD which he rented two days ago? So he grabs a refrigerated beer and a tub of microwaved pop corn, curls up on the sofa in front of the television, and, before he knows it, it is 2 A.M. And so the cycle repeats.

Apparently, the idea of "three regular meals every day" can easily be lost in a world full of emergencies and distractions. That will happen if we are not mindful about mundane activities like eating and rest. So what about if we place equal attention to work, eating and rest? What about if we plan and premeditate our eating plan as carefully as our career?

Do we really have to? The answer is yes, and you'd better do. Most people worry about getting fired if they cannot perform on the job. Along the same line of reasoning, if you don't eat properly, go to work with low energy, fail to concentrate and make an embarrassing mistake at work, you can also get fired. Your career can also suffer if you don't eat properly, become less resistant to diseases, catch the common flu from someone's coughs, and, instead of missing one day of work, have to stay

> **HABIT #14:**
> Pay equal attention to your work and eating habits — carefully plan for three well-balanced meals every day at regular, predictable times.

out of action for a whole week, miss the opportunity to take up the new project and miss the once-in-a-lifetime chance of getting promoted.

Well, if you are convinced to take your eating habits seriously, here are some important ideas to help you plan your meals.

(a) Breakfast

Breakfast is the most important meal of the day since the body's energy is focused on the key digestive organs during the morning hours (6 A.M. to 9 A.M.). In terms of cost effectiveness, this is the one meal that can be most efficiently digested and absorbed. Therefore, never skip breakfast just because you do not feel hungry.

Breakfast is the most important meal of the day as it sets the pace of your body's metabolism for the rest of the day.

Eat a well-balanced meal and eat enough food to fill the stomach to 100% of its capacity. Early in the morning, the body gauges its blood nutrient level and adjusts the overall metabolic rate accordingly for the day. That is why you will feel active, alert and focused (high metabolic rate) for the whole day if you eat a good breakfast, but sluggish and fuzzy (low metabolic rate) if you don't. In particular, if you are trying to lose weight, skipping breakfast is the worse possible way to achieve your goal — it will leave you with fat that refuse to burn off because your metabolic rate is so low all the time.

Good choices for a hearty breakfast include food in semi-liquid form, which are easy to digest and easy to absorb — such as hot cooked cereals, rice porridge and oatmeal. A soup noodle featuring cooked noodle or pasta, cooked meat and vegetables bathed in homemade broth is another of my favorite. For variety, eat a bun, toast, biscuit or egg sandwich (lightly scrambled egg served in a

> **HABIT #15:**
> For breakfast, avoid coffee, juice and fruit, but fill your stomach to 100% capacity with hot, easy-to-digest, semi-liquid food selections.

roll or between two pieces of bread), along with a hot nutritious drink, such as seed-based drinks and milk.

In any case, make sure you do not eat cold foods or drink cold liquid for breakfast. Therefore, avoid dry cereal with cold milk or cold soda — warm the milk and skip the soda. Do not eat fruit or drink fruit juice before noon as fruits purge the digestive system and cause the body to lose nutrients and moisture — save it for after lunch. Skip the coffee, too, as it is poor in nutrition and too much of a neural stimulant — replace it with a hot seed-based nutritious drink and feel the difference in genuine energy within your body. (I know this seems like a tall order, but all my patients who tried switching from coffee to a hot seed-based nutritious drink liked it and never went back to drinking coffee.)

(b) Lunch

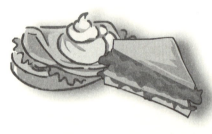

Lunch is your opportunity to relax and recuperate from your busy schedule.

Lunch time allows us to refuel and to recuperate before the afternoon activities. Do not hurry through it and do not work during lunch. It is best to take one hour in a pleasant environment, enjoy the tastes, textures and smells of the meal, and relax with your companions or in solitude. This is an opportunity to restore your mind and emotions, as well as you body.

You don't have to fill your stomach as much as in breakfast, but do eat to about 90% capacity of your stomach. To enhance digestion, eat a piece of fresh fruit (the size of an orange or apple; or equivalent amount of other fruits) at the end of lunch, but do not eat more than this moderate amount and do not eat chilled fruit.

Of course, when you choose the food items for lunch, don't forget the rules of "well-balanced meal" (Sect. 2-7) and "foods to avoid" (Sect. 2-10).

> HABIT #16:
> Eat lunch in a pleasant environment with a relaxed pace and finish with a small piece of fruit.

(c) Dinner

One important habit to ensure good digestion and good appetite for dinner is to avoid snacking, especially when it is near the expected dinner time. This is because most of the digestive juices, such as bile and pancreatic juices, are continuously made in small quantity throughout the day but are stored up, until the arrival of food, to be secreted in a large batch. When a person eats snacks, the small amount of food triggers the digestive system to deplete its reservoir of digestive juices prematurely, leading to a lack of digestive juices when the actual meal finally arrives. Furthermore, most of the common packaged snacks available tend to be highly processed and rich in sugar, which artificially elevates the blood sugar level, fooling the body into suppressing its own appetite during dinner.

Dinner is our chance to refuel before a restorative night's sleep.

As I have already mentioned, each meal, including dinner, should be eaten at a more-or-less fixed, predictable time. This is because, after one meal, the body has to take time to gear up for another round of ingestion and digestion — digestive juices have to be produced and accumulated, the stomach has to slowly return to an empty stage to initiate the hunger response, the duodenum has to clear its way, the pancreas has to sense a gradual fall of blood glucose level, hormones to increase appetite have to be gradually introduced, and the brain has to psychologically anticipate the pleasant experience of delicious food, etc. Needless to say, if you stick to a predictable eating schedule, your body will have an easier job coordinating these preparatory events to match the timing of the three daily meals.

> HABIT #17:
> Eat dinner at a *fixed, predictable time*, two to three hours before sleep, and avoid snacking before dinner time.

Dinner is the chance for us to refuel before a restorative night's sleep. Because our body, including the digestive system, will be going to a resting stage in a few hours after dinner, we want to give the digestive system enough time to complete the initial stages of digestion before we go to sleep. Therefore, fill the stomach only to 80% of its capacity and, as much as possible, finish the dinner before 8 P.M. After dinner, it is best to reduce eating and drinking to a minimum to allow the stomach and kidneys to rest when you sleep.

Of course, the rules of "well-balanced meal" (Sect. 2-7) and "foods to avoid" (Sect. 2-10) still apply for the dinner menu.

Sweet dessert following the evening meal is a Western tradition. The best choice (or substitute, depending on your perspective) for dessert is a piece of fresh fruit, which provides vitamins and fiber, and enhances the production of digestive enzymes. For a more traditional dessert, select items that are low in sugar and without stimulating spices such as cinnamon, and don't stuff yourself with sweet cakes — eat minimally for maximum enjoyment.

> HABIT #18:
> Eat a piece of fruit for dessert to enhance digestion and to avoid taking in unnecessary amount of sugar.

Sect. 2-12: Proper cooking methods

Even though I have already discussed the importance of avoiding raw and cold foods (Sect. 2-10(a) and (b)), I cannot overemphasize the importance of eating properly cooked foods. It is important to warm up our food by cooking so that, in order for the digestive enzymes to function optimally, we do not have to heat up the food with our own body heat and lose precious energy in the process. It is also very important to use cooking to pre-digest the matrix material of the food so that the nutrients can be readily released for absorption — uncooked vegetable has its vitamins trapped in the sap within the cellulose cell wall while uncooked pork is literally impenetrable by human teeth.

In TCM, cooking is also a way of neutralizing foods with extreme **energetic properties** (寒涼溫熱). TCM designates each kind of food with a certain energetic property — cold (寒), cool (涼),

neutral (中和), warm (溫) and hot (熱) — according to the way it affects the body medicinally. For example, most vegetables, fruits and fish are "**cool**", while pork and poultry are "**warm**"; seafood such as clams and oysters are "**cold**" while lamb and beef are "**hot**"; most carbohydrates, such as rice and pasta, are **neutral**.

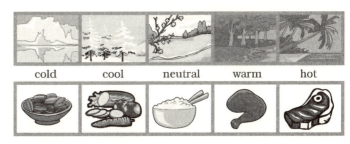

In TCM, different kinds of food are classified by their energetic properties, using the same language which we use to describe temperature. One of the objectives of cooking is to neutralize the foods that are too cold or too hot so that they will not energetically tilt our bodies out of balance.

So what exactly is the meaning of "hot" and "cold"? In general, "hot" foods are those that cause the body to display excessive metabolic activities, to become overheated and over-reactive. Thus tissues tend to become inflamed, membranes tend to lose moisture and become dry, nerves tend to spasm and joints tend to ache. "Warm" is simply a mild version of "hot".

On the other hand, "cold" foods have the exact opposite effects — they slow down general body functions and cause stagnation of substances within the tissues. Thus the membranes of the throat and bronchi accumulate mucus (resulting in coughing), the spleen cannot distribute nutrients efficiently, and a woman's uterus experiences menstrual difficulty. "Cool" is simply a mild version of "cold".

Indeed, this is the basis of Chinese herbal medicine. As an example, when a patient suffers from dehydration and constipation, his body's energetic state is diagnosed, by analysis of the pulse and tongue presentation, as being "hot". The TCM practitioner will prescribe herbs and foods that are energetically "cold" or "cool" to tip the patient back to a neutral state, thus curing the disease condition as the b alance is restored.

However, when vegetable and meat are to be consumed in large quantity as food, not as medicine, their intrinsic energetic properties are undesirable since we don't want to unwittingly push our body's energetic state off balance every time we eat. Therefore, when cooking foods that are not energetically neutral, we should use the appropriate ingredients to pre-neutralize them before they are served at the table. While this may be unheard of in Western culture, it is common knowledge to every Chinese family who does any amount of home cooking — for example, everybody knows to add several slices of ginger root (energetically warm) when cooking vegetable (energetically cool).

According to TCM, proper cooking methods are those that make food tastes delicious by (1) bringing out the natural flavor of the food while (2) preserving its nutrition and moisture content. This implies that cooking by intense heat, such as barbecue, grilling, charbroiling and deep frying, should be avoided because they tend to hurt the natural flavor and force out too much of the moisture content. It also means that we should avoid the use of heavy flavoring, such as thick dressings, overly salty or sweet sauces, hot sauces and spices, since they overwhelm the sense of taste and obliterate the natural flavor of the food.

Then what are proper cooking techniques that satisfy the TCM criteria? As we all know, the art of cooking itself can fill a huge volume. Therefore it is impossible to go into great details here without turning this book into a full-blown cookbook. Here I will only give suggestions and basic guidelines for cooking the three major food groups. (For readers who would like to learn more, I recommend my companion DVD and publications dedicated on healthy cooking techniques.)

> HABIT #19:
> Avoid cooking by intense heat (such as barbecue, grilling, charbroiling and deep frying) and the use of heavy flavoring (such as thick dressings, overly salty or sweet sauces, hot sauce and spices).

(a) Grains

White rice. The tricky part about cooking white rice is determining the correct ratio of rice grains and water, and the correct amount of time to cook — if slightly off, the rice will end up either too soggy or too dry. The easiest way around this problem is to cook white rice with an electric rice cooker, which has special marks in the pot as a guide for the proper water levels. The rest of the job is completely automatic — just plug in the power and press the button — the cooker will turn itself off when the rice is right.

Be sure to use regular rice, not the quick-cook or minute rice products that are highly processed and will not cook correctly in electric rice cooker.

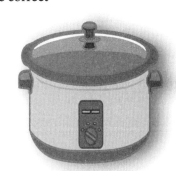

There is no easier way to cook white rice than to use an electric rice cooker.

Pasta. There is no trick to cooking pasta. Just add one teaspoonful of salt and one teaspoonful of oil into a pot of boiling water, then boil the spaghetti until soft. It takes about 8 minutes for spaghetti, less time for thinner pasta and more time for thicker one.

(b) Vegetables

Water cooking. (焯) This is the simplest and quickest way to cook vegetable. Add raw ginger root (2 slices), salt (1 tsp), sugar (½ tsp) and oil (1 tsp) into a pot of boiling water (8 to 10 cups). The ginger root neutralizes the cool property of the vegetable, while the salt and sugar bring out the natural flavor and color of the vegetable. Add the vegetable and stir to get all the greens under water.

The timing in the next step is critical. For lettuce, allow the vegetable to boil in the pot (open without lid) for 30 seconds and immediately remove the vegetable to a serving plate. For most other vegetables thicker than lettuce (e.g. spinach, broccoli), close the lid and allow to boil for 2 to 3 minutes (start timing only when steam emerges), then immediately remove the vegetable and drain off the water. If you like, serve the vegetable with soy sauce, oyster sauce or a dipping sauce.

The duration of boiling is critical as it is common for many people to boil much longer than necessary, resulting in the vegetable turning into a soggy green mush — the major complaint against water-cooked vegetable. It is also important not to leave the vegetable in the hot water when the boiling period is over since the vegetable will continue to be cooked by the heat, resulting, again, in a soggy green mush.

The secret to water cooking is to know the precise timing for each type of food cooked.

Stir-frying. (炒) This is a more complicated method than water boiling but results in a dish with a more stimulating and intense smell. Pre-heat two tsp. of oil in a wok or pan, stir in two slices of raw ginger root, then vigorously stir-fry the vegetable until the leaves turn darker green. Add salt (1 tsp) and sugar (½ tsp) and mix thoroughly; then after adding water to about 1 inch deep, cover the lid and let cook for 2 minutes (start timing only when steam emerges). After the 2 minutes, promptly open the lid and serve the vegetable on a plate.

Step 1: stir-fry

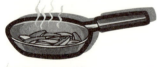

Step 2: cook with water

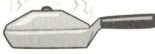

The secret to stir-frying is that it really is a two-step process and it is the cooking with water that preserve the flavor and moisture of the food.

The major benefit of stir-frying lies in the final step where the vegetable is further cooked with water — since the food does not have to be fully cooked by the stir-frying alone, the kind of intense heat used in grilling or deep frying is not necessary, resulting in much better preservation of the flavor and moisture content.

(c) Meat, poultry and fish

The quickest and easiest methods for cooking animal proteins are steaming and stir-frying, which are most suitable when you have only one hour or less before dinner must be ready to eat. However, if there is more time available to plan ahead, there is a large variety of cooking methods which can produce much more elaborated dishes, e.g. thermal pot cooking, stewing with Crock-Pots, poaching, pouch cooking, pressure cooking and covered baking in ceramic container or clay pot, etc. (For these more advanced cooking methods, please consult my companion DVD on healthy cooking.)

Steaming. (蒸) In this method, water at the bottom of a covered pot or wok is boiled into steam, which rises upward to indirectly cook a dish of meat elevated to just above the surface of the boiling water with a metal rack. This is the best method for preserving the natural flavor of the meat because the cooking temperature is at a modest 212°F (100°C) while the steam inside the pot prevents the moisture content of the food from escaping. Any "juice" that emerge from the meat is caught in the dish, which can be used as a sauce.

This method is particularly suitable for fish, the flesh of which is delicate and can easily fall apart with too much handling in other cooking methods. I also use steaming for cooking chunks of chicken, minced pork, ribs (pre-cut to one-inch dices) and homogenized eggs (pre-diluted with two times water by volume).

Before steaming, the meat or poultry should be cut into bite-size pieces or thin slices. Then the pieces have to be marinated with salt and sugar, then with corn starch and finally with oil

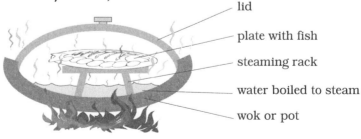

For steaming, a wok is the best choice for the outside container since it is wide and shallow, allowing even a large plate to be placed inside. The steaming rack, as well as a special claw-like tool for lifting the plate into and out of the wok, can be purchased from most Chinese kitchen supply stores.

— all of which enhance the natural flavors and neutralizes the energetic property of the meat. On the other hand, fish can be steamed whole and without marinating if soy sauce is to be used after steaming for flavoring. In order to neutralize the cool property, however, fish should be steamed after being topped with ginger root slices or strips.

Add water into a pot or wok to 2 inches deep. Place a metal steaming rack in the pot, making sure that the top of the rack is well above the water surface. Close the lid and boil the water with high power. When steam emerges, open the lid and place the dish of the marinated meat on top of the rack. Close the lid and make sure it closes tightly (but not air-tight) — if it doesn't, you'll need a bigger pot or a lower steaming rack. When steam emerges once again, turn the fire power to medium-high and start timing.

As a first trial, steam for 3 minutes for homogenized egg, 5 minutes for fish, and 10 minutes for pork and chicken. When the time is up, open the lid and test if the meat has been fully cooked by poking a chopstick into it — if has been fully cooked, you should be able to penetrate through without much resistance. Steam for extra minutes if it is not fully cooked yet.

Stir-frying. (炒) The process of stir-frying meat and poultry is very similar to stir-frying vegetable. In fact, I usually stir-fry some sliced or diced meat immediately after I finish stir-frying some vegetable — so that the two can be combined into one dish. Thus, in one single dish, I have enough food to take care of two of the three food groups in a meal.

There are a few minor differences when stir-frying meat, however. First, the seasoning is introduced into the meat by marinating (with salt and sugar, then with corn starch, then with oil) before the stir-frying. No additional salt or sugar is necessary during or after stir-frying.

A kitchen's best friends: green onion (to cook with meat and beef) and ginger root (to cook with vegetables and fish). They are suitable for all kinds of cooking methods, especially stir-frying, water cooking and steaming.

Second, when stir-frying meat or poultry, we use green onion leaves (cut to one-inch segments; discard the very bottom end with the roots) instead of ginger root slices to initiate the stir-frying. Green onion has the appearance of a slim version of leek (unlike the spherical yellow onion), and is good for neutralizing the warm property of meat and poultry. However, for stir-frying fish, which is energetically cool, continue to use ginger root as in stir-frying vegetable.

Third, after stir-frying, you also add water to 2 inches deep and cover the pot to further steam cook the meat with medium fire power — but the cooking duration is longer than with vegetable because meat is usually thicker and tougher. Try 4 minutes for your first attempt. The one exception is beef, usually cut into thin slices, as it should not be further steam cooked after stir-frying — for some reason, its texture will become very tough if you do.

Fourth, at the end of the additional steam-cooking, you will have accumulated some sauce derived from the meat in the pot — it is customary to turn it into a gravy to enhance the flavor. To make a gravy, thoroughly pre-mix a quarter teaspoonful of salt and sugar, two teaspoonful of cornstarch and three soup spoonful of water, then stir in the slurry to the sauce at the bottom of the wok or pan. Continue to stir the liquid gently with the fire still on and watch the sauce turns into a thicker gravy. Immediately turn off the fire when you have the right thickness for the gravy.

Some of you may want to see the above techniques demonstrated before trying them in your own kitchen. Some of you may be eager to learn more advanced techniques and tips to cook delicious and healthy meals. In either case, I urge you to check out my companion DVD on healthy cooking for further information.

> HABIT #20:
> Use proper cooking methods, such as water-cooking, steaming and stir-frying, to bring out the natural flavors while preserving the nutrition and moisture content of food.

Sect. 2-13: Practical tips for eating out

It should be apparent that home-cooked meals made from fresh, unprocessed and nutritious ingredients provide the maximum benefits in the acquisition of vital substance. But as we have to occasionally dine out, we are once again beckoned by grilled food, barbecued food, deep-fried food, spicy food, raw food, cold food, heavily-flavored food, cold drinks and alcoholic beverages. Is there anything we can do about this?

The key to dining out is to think warm, nutritious and balanced. You are likely to have to ask extra questions and make extra requests. But don't be afraid — most restaurants which pride themselves of catering to the individual needs of the customers will be happy to abide — in the hope for customer's loyalty and extra tips. It actually works both ways.

Here are a few tips (of the non-monetary kind) that I can offer.

Ice water. The waiter brings it, often without asking, and sets the tinkling glasses on the table, dripping with condensation. But you don't have to drink it — and no one will notice. Or you can ask for water without ice before the waiter leaves.

In many restaurants, the waiter will ask if you want water anyway. That will be the perfect time to request "no ice". On an airplane, I always request "no ice please" when the flight attendant ask me what I like to drink. Why wouldn't you? You get more drink in your tiny plastic cup and no ice to numb your gum.

Hot drink before eating. Order a cup of hot tea (non-caffeinated tea, such as herbal tea) before you order the meal so you can start warming up your digestive tract. You can dip the herbal tea bag in the hot water for a mild brew, or just drink the hot water. After the meal, ask for a refill of hot water for your tea as a cleansing drink.

Another alternative is to order a hot soup and request that it be served before the main course. In Chinese

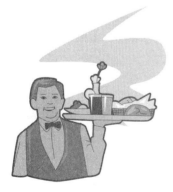

Good waiters pride themselves of serving the customers. So don't hesitate to make special requests and ask extra questions of your waiter.

restaurants, you can order a jumbo-sized bowl of soup to be shared by everyone at the table.

Entree selection. You want to put together an order that includes all three food groups — grains, vegetables and meats. In addition, you also want to avoid spicy, cold and raw dishes.

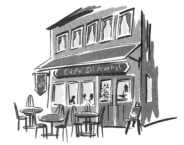

Do you know if your favorite restaurants offer health-compatible dishes or take special orders?

Many restaurant menus specifically marked their spicy dishes with asterisks or icons of chili pepper — avoid those. If you do like a certain dish except for the spice, ask if they can, for example, prepare the sirloin steak without the pepper rub. This question often reveals whether the restaurant prepares the food in a big batch in advance or individually on ordering (which means it is fresh from the stove).

If the spicy dishes are not clearly marked in the menu and the spices are not listed in the entree description, take the time to ask the waiter for the ingredients.

Instead of a raw salad, ask if the kitchen can take a special order for cooked vegetables, rice or potato. Or, instead of deep-fried selections, ask if they can prepare a simple pan-fried cut of meat.

If there are no suitable entrees and a special order is not possible, order a number of side dishes to put together a makeshift meal, such as English muffin or toast, a scrambled egg and a glass of hot milk.

Of course, when you finally identify restaurants that are capable of offering health-compatible dishes or taking special orders, patronize them and praise their individualized service.

Potlucks. With total uncertainty of the kinds of food you will find, the best strategy is to bring a dish that meets your dietary needs. Be sure to bring enough to share and provide yourself with a full meal, just in case.

> HABIT #21:
> *Take appropriate measures when eating out to maintain good eating habits and to avoid foods that harm our health.*

Otherwise, choose as best you can from the dishes available. Remember, it is what we eat on a daily basis that builds our health and eating an occasional spaghetti sauce with garlic or a raw green leafy salad with a vinaigrette dressing will not necessarily cause permanent damage to your health.

Meals prepared by family and friends. While family and friends want to nourish us with lovingly prepared meals, these traditional meals often contain ingredients that tax the body, such as garlic and pepper, or are cooked with methods that do not preserve well the nutrients and moisture content of the food.

However, being part of a family or circle of friends also includes being interested in what each other is doing and in accommodating each other's needs and goals. Therefore, don't be shy to talk openly about the new health path you are taking and they will usually support your efforts at the dinner table. You can also help make your point by bringing an entree that meets your needs.

There will be occasions when the food being served is not health-compatible, such as a piece of overly sweetened birthday cake. But as long as you know your limits and your daily diet is healthy, there is no need to be over-alarmed by an occasional exception.

X   X   X

In this chapter, we have taken a long journey through the digestive system of our bodies, through the aisles of the supermarkets, through the kitchens and the restaurants, and even through the life of a typical modern-day worker. It has taken quite a bit of effort to learn the strategies necessary to become a skillful energy investor.

But as many hard-working people might have already known, the monthly paycheck you receive can quickly evaporate after the bills are paid, leaving nothing behind to be saved for a new house or for emergency needs. You will soon find out, just as it is important to earn vital substance, it is equally important to control your expenditures so that you can build up the much needed vital essence, necessary for unforeseen events and for self-healing. That will be our topic in the next chapter.

80

CHAPTER 3
CONSERVING VITAL FORCE

Sect. 3-1: The global consequences of energy debt
- (a) Chronic fatigue
- (b) Digestive problems
- (c) Insomnia
- (d) Hot flashes
- (e) Weak immune system
- (f) Muscle and tendon injuries
- (g) Negative mental and emotional states
- (h) Return of old symptoms
- (i) Weight gain

Sect. 3-2: Activities that interfere with resting
- (a) Nighttime activity
- (b) Inadequate breaks

Sect. 3-3: Over-exercising

Sect. 3-4: Intensified mental and emotional states

Sect. 3-5: Unnecessary heat loss
- (a) Weather conditions
- (b) Direct contact
- (c) Breathing dry or damp air
- (d) Faulty washing habits
- (e) Highly-contrasting indoor and outdoor temperatures
- (f) Eating cold food and drink

Sect. 3-1: The global consequences of energy debt

As we have discussed in Chapter 1 (Sect. 1-6), one of the most important strategies to achieve good health is to build a strong reserve of vital essence — the energy "savings" that keeps our body from faltering in adverse and emergency situations. Thus, in the context of SAVINGS = DEPOSIT – WITHDRAWAL, we have discussed the many ways we can increase our "savings" by maximizing our "deposit" of daily energy intake. Now we will turn our attention to the second half of the equation — how we can minimize our "withdrawal".

The proposal to minimize withdrawal of energy, however, creates a kind of conundrum for us. If all we care is to spend the minimum amount of energy in our daily life, of course, the easiest way would be to sit still and do as little as possible. But, unless we are monks living in a monastery, that is rather incompatible with life in a modern society, which requires us to stay active and competitive throughout the day. How do we resolve the simultaneous needs to conserve and consume energy?

This situation commonly occurs whenever we have limited resources — water, electricity, money, time, etc. When water conservation is enforced during a drought, no one is being asked not to wash and not to drink — you are simply asked to wash and drink less so as not to exhaust the water available. When parents ask children to conserve their money, they are not telling them to stop spending completely — but just not to buy so much that the allowance completely disappears.

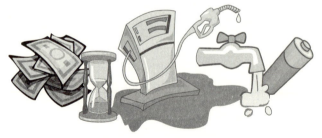

What does vital substance have in common with money, time, gasoline, water and battery power? They are all limited resources that we cannot afford to run out of.

So perhaps we need to clarify exactly what we want to achieve here. When we say we should minimize the spending of vital force, we mean that we want to lead an active life while still staying within the energy budget available to us. Thus, we can still consume vital substance, but just not so much or so fast that our energy output

(WITHDRAWAL) exceeds our energy intake (DEPOSITS) — a situation we call **energy debt**.

This sounds fine, but that creates yet another problem. When we are consuming too much water in a dry year, the city's water department will issue warning reports about our reservoirs running dry. When we are spending too much and writing too many checks, we will receive a bank statement showing a rapidly-decreasing account balance to warn us that we are running out of money. But who is going to warn us if our body is consuming vital substance beyond its energy budget?

Just imagine what happens to your body in a crisis situation — your project report is due tomorrow and you must stay up all night to finish it. Your brain must stay alert even after it exhausts its daily ration of vital substance. It has just entered the state of energy debt and so it taps into its storage of vital essence to keep itself going.

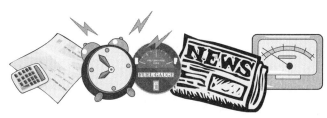

Bank statement, alarm clock, fuel gauge, newspaper report and battery tester are tools that help monitor those other limited resources and warn us when their levels go too low. But what tool can we use to monitor the level of our vital substance?

Now let's prolong the scenario — you have to stay up for *three* consecutive nights to finish. Your brain soon exhausts all its vital essence and, in order to keep on working, your body starts shifting vital essence from other organs with less urgent needs to supply the brain. Before long, these "other organs", usually those that provide background maintenance services, will begin to show signs of failing.

These "signs of failing" are the signs of energy debt — the warning signals that tell us that we are spending way too much energy than is available. They do not come from someone or somewhere else but your own body, so you have to constantly monitor yourself for them. A lot of times, these signs are subtle and unless you pay close attention

> The signs of energy debt come from your own body and are often subtle. Unless you pay close attention to your body, you may miss them all together.

to your body, you may miss them all together. So how do I know when I am experiencing the signs of energy debt?

To be sure, your brain itself will experience fatigue, just as a toy train starts failing to climb an incline when the battery begins to run out. But the most significant feature of the signs of energy debt is that they happen globally — liver, kidney, stomach, immune system, skin, sexual organs, etc. — even in organs remotely related with the brain. They are putting off their normal functions as their reserves of vital essence have been taken away.

Here are some common examples of signs of energy debt:

(a) Chronic fatigue

Fatigue is the feeling for the need to rest. This is the way the brain tells you that its battery is running out of power for the day and that it needs to stop working until more vital substance can be acquired and sent to the brain. We often feel fatigue at the end of a hard day of work and it can be treated simply with good food and some extra sleep. This type of temporary fatigue is quite normal and nothing to be worried about, since the energy level should bounce back to normal the next morning.

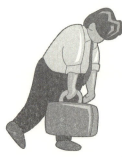

If you continue to feel tired after waking up in the morning, you are in a state of chronic fatigue.

What is to be worried is the chronic type of fatigue that does not go away even after a night's sleep. Instead you continue to feel tired after waking up in the morning, your energy level fluctuates in and out of tiredness throughout the day and your mind has a hard time concentrating on the task at hand. Without further thought, many people will just reach for a cup of coffee to douse the ongoing fatigue — little do they know that it is a warning that their energy debt is much more serious than what one normal sleep cycle can restore and they are running on an empty fuel tank.

In TCM, this condition is known as "**phantom flame**" (虛火). The closest analogy is that of a teapot (the body) that has been boiling for so long that all its water (vital essence) has evaporated while the flame still continues to burn. While the teapot has become overheated, the flame is not producing any steam (chi) at all — it is nothing more than a "futile flame".

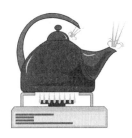

If the water in a teapot disappears due to prolonged boiling (energy debt), not only will you run out of steam (chronic fatigue), you will also be left with an overheated teapot (hot flash).

(b) Digestive problems

When the vital essence is taken away from the digestive system, it begins to run out of power and show signs of sluggishness and inefficiencies — indigestion, heartburn, gas, cold stomach (feel the area of the skin over the stomach), constipation and diarrhea. It is no use to reach for medicine for heartburn or gas or constipation, because there is really nothing wrong with the digestive system itself. You will not find any abnormality when the stomach, intestine or liver are examined with X-ray and lab tests — yet the digestive problems persist.

This reminds me of a friend who asked me to fix her computer because "the hard disk is not working". When I arrived, I found that the hard disk indeed failed to spin up and my friend went into panic when I mumbled that the hard disk might have crashed ("Oh, no! I didn't backup the files!"). But, as it turned out, the power cord that supplied the hard disk was simply loosened — upon my firm plugging in, the whole computer sprung back to life!

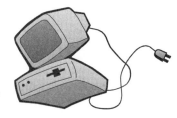

And that's how the digestive system feels like when the body goes into energy debt — it is capable of doing work but it cannot due to lack of power. The stomach, liver, pancreas and intestine are slow to produce digestive juices.

When your organ systems appear to have fallen ill due to energy debt, they are no more broken than a computer that has been unplugged.

The pH's of the different regions go out of range. Peristalsis becomes sluggish and so is absorption of water and nutrients. The digestive system appears to have caught some major disease — but not really, it just needs power.

(c) Insomnia

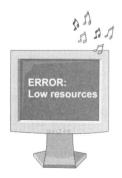

Late into the night, you are very, very tired. So why can't you fall asleep?

This is probably one of the biggest paradoxes for people who overworked. They are so tired that they keep nodding off during the day. Yet, when they finally get the chance to go to bed, they are on their back with eyes wide open, unable to fall asleep. Others fall asleep initially, but then wake up in the middle of the night with sweat over the body (see part (d) "Hot flashes") unable to fall back to sleep — giving rise to the infamous expression "wide awake at 3 A.M." (There is even a book on sleep disorder with this exact title)

Well, remember (from Sect. 1-8) that the sleeping period is the time when our organs carry out their daily maintenance work — the patching up and reconditioning from all the wear and tear received during the day? Remember that the energy required for this self-healing process comes from the vital essence? If our body is in a state of energy debt and vital essence is low, the organs will have difficulties finishing the self-regeneration process and, in response, they start sending "error messages" to the brain.

When a computer runs into an error, it pauses everything, makes an annoying "ding" sound and flashes an unsightly error message — all this to catch your attention.

As a result, the brain is continuously interrupted by these "blips and bops" from what should have been quiet automatic background processes throughout the night — and that is why it cannot sleep peacefully. In fact, such a person often wakes up more than once during the night, often around the transition times when the energy moves from one organ to the next (i.e. 1 A.M., 3 A.M., 5 A.M., etc.) (more details in Sect. 5-2) — when a whole new set of "error messages" are emitted by a new organ.

Again, it is no use to reach for the tranquilizer or sleeping pill. For a few years in the mid 1990s, a pill made of melatonin, a natural hormone which triggers sleepiness, became the fashionable panacea for insomnia — and then dropped out of fashion again. Why? Because all these chemicals are ineffective for the same reason — they act on the brain but there is nothing wrong with the brain. The body is simply in energy debt.

(d) Hot flashes (night sweats)

Although commonly associated with women undergoing menopause, hot flashes also occur in pre-menopausal women and men who experience a state of energy debt. When hot flash occurs, the heart rate increases, the blood pressure goes up, the blood vessels dilate, a feeling of heat flush through the body surface, and the body sweats profusely. When this happens during sleep, the person often wakes up with the clothes and pillow soaking wet with sweat — often when the room temperature is not hot, or even warm.

Why are these happening? These physiological responses are very much like those that occur when one goes into a hot environment, such as a sauna, and the body tries hard to cool itself to a lower temperature. But in hot flash, the heat does not come from the external environment — rather, the heat originates from the "phantom flame" that occurs internally due to the absence of vital essence (see the earlier discussion under "(a) Chronic fatigue"). The heart, blood vessels, skin and sweat glands are completely normal — they are simply responding naturally to the "heat" within the body, which has run into severe energy debt.

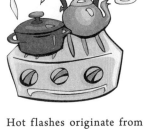

Hot flashes originate from the internal "phantom flame" during energy debt, just as teapots become overheated when they carry no more water to receive the heat of the stove.

(e) Weak immune system

When a person overwork, much energy has to be channeled away from organs performing less urgent functions — notably those of the immune system. One way in which the body does this is to command the adrenal glands to secrete stress hormones called adrenocorticosteroids, which sustain a high-alert state (high blood pressure, high blood glucose level) and simultaneously suppress the immune system. In fact, adrenocorticosteroids (e.g. cortisol) are so strongly immunosuppressive that modified forms of these hormones are used medicinally to suppress inflammation in skin rashes and in rheumatoid arthritis (e.g. cortisone).

Remember, in Sect. 1-2, I (H.L.) mentioned how I always seemed to catch the flu when I overextended my work days as a high-school teacher? When the immune system weakens as energy is channeled away to organs with more urgent needs, you find yourself falling to some mundane illnesses such as cold and flu, which you normally can resist quite well. Even before falling ill, you may experience prolonged period of a vague foggy-headed feeling, physical weakness, irritability, congestive airways, vivid dreams and fatigue.

A little headache, stuffy nose or sore throat may be minor discomforts, but they reflect a sluggish immune system about to give way to real diseases.

Again, there is nothing wrong with your immune system — they are just being put on standby mode. If you are experiencing the early warnings of illness, you may still be able to minimize the effects of the illness by immediately getting more rest and eating easy-to-digest food to replenish the vital essence.

(f) Muscle and tendon injuries

When a person is in energy debt, the normal self-healing process, which requires vital essence, has to be put on hold. Thus, the daily wear and tear of muscles and tendons cannot be promptly and properly repaired. Over time, the dilapidated muscles and tendons become very vulnerable to injury — even by what is considered gentle motions, such as putting on a jacket or bending down to tie the shoelaces.

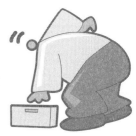

Being prone to physical injury is a sign that your body's tissues have been poorly maintained.

These energy-debt injuries happen easily and are different from injuries caused by overexertion, such as lifting a heavy object or pulling weeds for four hours. Of course, when the muscle or tendon injury happens, it has to be treated promptly and properly. But unless the energy debt situation is resolved at the same time, the patient will easily experience another episode of injury or simply re-injure himself.

(g) Negative mental and emotional states

You have no doubt met someone who came to work in a bad mood because of the stress over work and the lack of sleep. When a person is in the state of energy debt, multiple organ systems of the body begin to malfunction, causing him to experience general discomfort and irritability. At this stage, the mind becomes preoccupied with negative thoughts and feelings, such as anxiety, frustration, edginess, resentment, anger and fear — which can cause additional drain on the body's vital essence as they intensify, further aggravating the energy debt situation.

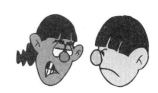

The discomfort due to failure of multiple organs makes people grouchy and irritable.

Therefore, pay attention to your thoughts and feelings — they are the barometer for your body's energy state. In addition, when negative thoughts and feelings occur, don't reach out for mood-altering drugs, such as cigarette, alcohol, marijuana and other recreational drugs. What you really need is more vital essence — more energy input and less energy output.

(h) Return of old symptoms

During times of energy debt, it is common for old symptoms from previous health conditions to return, even those that have fully recovered. This is because organs weakened by prior illness are likely to need extra maintenance and reconditioning through the daily self-regeneration process in order to continue to function normally. Thus, when this self-regeneration process is interrupted by the effect of low vital essence, these organs are often the first ones to exhibit problems.

(i) Weight gain

A lot of people think that weight gain is purely a dietary problem. Thus when weight gain occurs, many people switch to a low-calorie / low-carb / low-fat / low-protein / low-everything weight-loss diet or resort to vigorous sweat-producing exercise to "burn the fat". Nonetheless, even though some people initially experience temporary weight loss, the body fails to lose weight in the long term and, instead, continues to gain weight. Why?

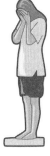

Sudden weight gain, especially when there has been no significant change in diet or physical activities, is indicative of chemical imbalance in your body.

According to TCM, as long as a healthy person is eating a balanced diet, his body should be able to utilize the nutrients from food and eliminate any excess nutrients as metabolic wastes — which means a healthy, active adult is automatically capable of preventing himself from gaining weight. But if the body enters a state of energy debt, many of the less urgent, background maintenance functions have to be put on hold — among them, (you guessed it!) the elimination of excess nutrients and metabolic wastes performed by the liver and kidneys. Thus these undesirable materials accumulate in the body and much of them are converted or incorporated into fatty tissue to be secluded from other tissues.

Just imagine what happened to your home when you were too busy to attend to household chores — didn't you find dirty dishes stacking up in the sink, food scraps scattering all over the dinner table, waste paper flying over the floor, dirty clothes spilling from the laundry basket, litter bins overflowing with garbage, and trash cans failing to be hauled out for collection? In short, the home seems to be bursting at the seams with wastes of one kind or another! This is how the body is like when the background job of cleaning up is put on hold during the crisis of energy debt.

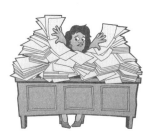

A desk overflowing with unwanted papers — a sure sign that someone has been too busy to clean up the desk.

Even worse, going on diet likely means taking in a less-than-sufficient amount of nutritious food as required by a normal, active person. Thus the digestive system will obtain even less vital substance than before, further reducing the amount of vital essence the body can save up. The body will sink ever deeper into the state of energy debt.

x   x   x

By now, it should be amply clear that entering energy debt can cause widespread harmful effects on many parts of the body — so much so that the causes of many of the common ailments listed in the opening section of this book (Sect. 1-1) have been explained in this section by energy debt alone. Unfortunately, many patients make the mistake of focusing on the one organ involved in a particular ailment, be it the lower back in muscle injury or the brain in insomnia, while failing to realize that the real cause lies in a much more general category — faulty living habits that overspend vital force.

It is very important that you pay close attention to your body and monitor for the common signs of energy debt — and immediately make adjustments to your living habits to ease the energy debt crisis. However, we do not have

> HABIT #22:
> Pay close attention to your body for signs of energy debt. When they occur, instead of just reaching into the drug cabinet for quick fixes of the symptoms, immediately make adjustments to your living habits to ease the energy debt crisis.

to wait for signs of energy debt to occur before making adjustments to your living habits to conserve vital force. In the following sections, I will discuss many common mistakes in our daily life which often lead to unnecessary overspending of vital force. Pay attention to any of these mistakes that apply to you and make plan to correct them proactively.

Sect. 3-2: Activities that interfere with resting

Many of my career-conscious patients feel a little guilty when I tell them that the body needs time to *rest* as much as it needs time to *work*. Although the body appears externally to be idle when resting, the fact is that it continues to work very hard internally, but in a quiet and invisible way — it refocuses its energy on functions related to background maintenance, such as digestion, immune response, elimination of wastes, tissue repair and reconditioning. Therefore, if a person extend his external activities into the period when the body expects to rest, a conflict of energy allocation will occur, leading to low efficiencies of both external and internal functions.

(a) Nighttime activity

The night hours between 10:30 P.M. and 6:30 A.M. are crucial for the daily recharging cycle because this is the time when the body instinctively channels its energy to the internal organs important to digestive health, especially the liver and gall bladder (see Chapter 5 for details). Therefore if a person forces himself to engage in physical, mental or emotional activity during this period, he will have to pay an extra overhead cost to re-channel the energy back to the brain and muscles from the internal organs. Thus the total energy

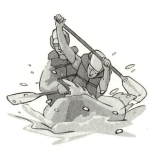

If you have to travel by canoe, will you choose to do so at a time when the current is against you?

needed during nighttime could end up being several times the energy needed to perform the same action during the day.

As a way to visualize this phenomenon, imagine that you want to row a canoe downstream into the bay. This is best done during ebb tide when the current flows from the river towards the bay, carrying your canoe in the same direction of your travel. However, if you insist on traveling downstream during the flood tide when the current is flowing upstream, you will have to spend several times more energy to row against the current before you can reach your downstream destination. Similarly, if you are to perform a mental or physical action during nighttime, you will be wasting tremendous amount of energy since the direction of energy flow is unfavorable to the brain and muscles.

Sometimes we have to extend our daytime activities into the night due to necessity — such as overtime work, night shift, or a rush to meet a deadline. These situations should really be kept to a minimum with better planning ahead of time, including frank negotiations with teammates and boss, if necessary. You will likely perform more efficiently and achieve better result if you consistently do your work when your body is most suited to support external activities.

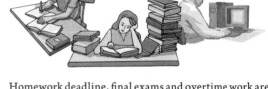

Homework deadline, final exams and overtime work are some of the occasions when we have to work grudgingly into the night.

Some people accept nighttime jobs by choice for a chance to earn more money, which seems to be harder and harder to come by in these days of frequent downsizing. In this case, you will have to make the judgment as to how much good health is worth to you. When you do so, keep these in mind — first, money is not very useful when you do not have the health to enjoy it; second, as you pass the age of 40, your body becomes less and less resilient and, before long, no amount of money can buy you health.

> HABIT #23:
> In order to utilize your energy more cost-effectively, avoid extending daytime work activities into late evening with better time management.

Ultimately, your wealth will be measured by your health, not by your money.

Other people choose to participate in "nightlife" activities for the sake of fun or entertainment — going out for parties, drinks, discos, night clubs or movies, playing games or just watching TV late into the wee hours at home. These activities seem to be fun since we are stimulated and oblivious to the internal signals from our bodies — but when the excitement disappears, we feel the pain of not having allowed the body to rest when rest was needed. As our age advances, the toll on the body will become more and more noticeable.

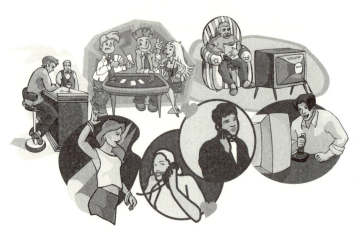

Disco dancing, night bar, gaming with friends, late night TV shows, video games, marathon phone chats: a few examples of how people spend their late evening time for entertainment.

For these situations, my advice would be to start your activity early and finish it before 9:30 P.M. when it is still fun without punishing your body. If this arrangement does not allow enough time for your activity, schedule them during daytime on a weekend or a holiday when you are off from work. If the idea of partying or watching movies during the day does not appeal to you, you might want to rethink your idea of fun and find some other activities you can enjoy during the day.

HABIT #24:
Avoid late-night entertainments which prevent the body from receiving proper rest when rest is needed.

(b) Inadequate breaks.

Besides the long sleep at night, it is also important for us to take rest breaks periodically during the day — typically one ten-minute break every two hours. These breaks are necessary because, like an engine running at full speed, our body spends vital force as a foreground task much faster than it can acquire vital substance as a background task. The short breaks are needed to allow the body to momentarily shift its focus to the organs responsible for energy acquisition so that the recharging process can be accelerated to catch up with the spending.

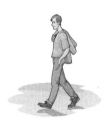

If you usually work at the desk, take a short walk for your ten-minute break.

Thus, during the day, if you neglect to take ten-minute breaks periodically, or continue to work while eating lunch at your desk, or maintain a tightly-packed schedule of constant activities, you run the risk of exhausting your deposit of vital substance and ending up in energy debt.

It is interesting how many of my patients try to bargain with me when I tell them to take a ten-minute break every two hours. At this point, I simply point out that my laptop computer requires two hours of recharging for every two hours of operation under battery power. If you think about it, a ten-minute break is not so bad for a "machine" as active, massive and complicated as your body.

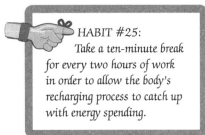

HABIT #25:
Take a ten-minute break for every two hours of work in order to allow the body's recharging process to catch up with energy spending.

Sect. 3-3: Over-exercising

It seems to be a very popular belief among white-collar workers and students that good health can best be achieved through regular sweat-producing workouts, sometimes coupled with a low-calorie or low-carb diet (thus the term "keep fit", which has the dual meaning of "staying healthy" and "staying thin"). I have met many people who

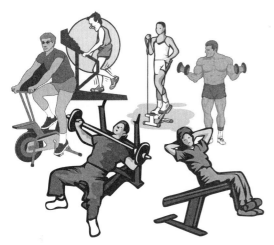

Perhaps due to the recent fitness craze, the above image has become a familiar evening scene in fitness centers around the city.

would run to the fitness gym every day to fulfill an hour-long exercise regime on a treadmill or stationary bike, even when it is late in the evening after putting in a full day of work. Others would jog for miles along the roadside in the early morning hours before showering and heading to work, adding fitness exercise to their already packed work and personal schedules.

Very often, it actually feels good to work up a sweat as strenuous exercises can induce a feeling of euphoria by stimulating the secretion of endorphins and other neurotransmitters of pleasure in the brain. In addition, the media and magazines out there constantly remind us that exercising is good for preventing high blood pressure, heart disease, obesity, diabetes, respiratory disease, depression, etc., and for strengthening muscles, bones, joints and the immune system. So what could possibly go wrong with exercising?

The trouble is that these messages are meant for the very young people who have plenty of energy to spare and can bounce back to their hyperactive condition in a heartbeat — which reminds me of teenagers, who seem to be constantly screaming and running around all day long. It probably applies to many college students in their late teens and early twenties, too. But if you are old enough to have a regular job, pay your bills, build a romantic relationship, care for your family, manage your home, do household chores and have numerous other tiresome responsibilities, then you no longer have boundless energy and daily strenuous exercise is probably not right for you.

The fact is that how much exercise and what kind of exercise is appropriate vary from person to person, depending on the age, workload, health history, physical condition and state of energy savings. Keep in mind that the energy expense on fitness exercise is in addition to the energy already spent on work, family and self-care. From my clinical experience, a daily one-hour vigorous workout regime is, in fact, overtaxing for the typical adult with a full-time job.

Another problem is with performing strenuous exercise in the evening, i.e. after 6:00 P.M., which is often the case for people who work out after work. At this time, our body should be allowed to relax and slowly transition to the yin (or resting) state in preparation for sleep. But if we are to exercise vigorously at this time, we will artificially postpone the body's preparation for sleep and may find ourselves unable to fall asleep peacefully at bedtime — thus interfering with the nightly self-healing process.

> HABIT #26:
> *Do not overexert yourself with strenuous exercise if you have a full-time workload or if the time has already passed 6 P.M.*

The key to health-promoting exercise is to do it with moderation — there is no point in force-feeding your body with demanding exercises that your body cannot afford to do. So, instead of sweat-producing workouts, what alternatives do we have? Believe it or not, there are plenty of such moderate activities that do not overtax our body — we just do not usually associate them with exercising.

Try looking for practical exercises, especially those around the home. Mow the lawn, tend the yard (instead of hiring a gardener), rake the leaves, sweep the deck, mop the floor, pull the weeds of the driveway, clean out the cob webs, vacuum the carpets, wash the windows, clear out the rain gutters, wash the car, bathe the dog, do the laundry, play with the kids, reorganize the shelves, change the bed sheets — most household chores are light workout opportunities that will

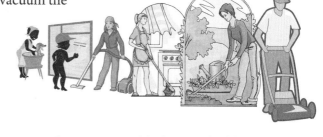

Practical exercises around the house are less likely to drain your energy as strenuous exercises do: (from left to right) bathe the dog, wash the windows, vacuum the carpet, sweep the floor, tend the garden, mow the yard, etc.

not break your back. What's more — you can enjoy the result of your "exercise" when you are done.

Try giving yourself chances for some gentle exercise. Park your car a few blocks from work and walk to the office, ride a bike to work instead of driving, take a walk at lunch or during a break, or take the stairs instead of riding the elevator. Go for a swim but, instead of racing to break someone's record, do it gently to enjoy the motion and rhythm of your strokes. Go for a walk on a nature trail but, instead of running for your life, take the time to enjoy the sight, sound and smell, and observe the changes of the season. Take a dance class with a friend or spouse and enjoy the artistic aspect of your exercise.

Walking to work, chi gong exercise, walking the dog, riding the bicycle to school (left to right): these are some gentle exercises that can be enjoyed by people of all ages.

There is one other possibility which may have never crossed your mind — chi-enhancing exercise, the most well-known form being **chi gong** (or qi gong, 氣功). This is a light-weight exercise that incorporates movements and postures specifically designed to strengthen the flow of chi through the meridians (see Sect. 1-7) You can think of chi gong as a TCM-based physical therapy that simultaneously gives you the dual benefits of exercising and therapy (see Chapter 4 for details) — so you get two things done at the same time. In fact, it is so popular in China that numerous people, young and old, can be seen practicing chi gong every day wherever there are public parks.

HABIT #27:
Replace strenuous exercises with practical exercises around the house or gentle exercises that do not overtax your body.

Sect. 3-4: Intensified mental and emotional states

As a survival mechanism, our bodies are physiologically wired to respond with a set of rapid reactions called the "fight-or-flight responses" whenever we are faced with life-threatening danger, sometimes even before we are consciously aware of the danger itself. This is what happens when you are walking alone down a long, quiet hallway and, all of a sudden, someone taps on your shoulder. Immediately you jump, rapidly turn around and possibly scream — but even after you find out it was just your old friend trying to surprise you, you can still feel your blood racing, your heart banging loudly and rapidly, your chest heaving up and down to catch the breath, your head sweating profusely, your eyes wide open, and your adrenaline rushing — as if you have just run the 100-meter dash.

This kind of response is most helpful when facing actual, dangerous situations, such as a car accident, violent crime or a burning house, since it shortens our response time, heightens our alertness and prepares us for vigorous physical action. But the "fight-or-flight response" does take a toll on our bodies since a huge amount of energy must be consumed to accelerate the full range of vital functions — which is why we feel totally drained even long after an episode of imminent threat. To be sure, unless absolutely necessary, we want to avoid putting ourselves routinely in such an exhausting situation.

When a person faces imminent danger, such as a ferocious animal in hot pursuit, the "fight-or-fright responses" will kick-start his body to either fight against or run away from the danger.

However, while our bodies can be triggered to display the "fight-or-flight responses" by *real* dangerous threats, they can also be easily tricked into displaying similar responses by *imaginary* threats, even when we consciously recognize the threats to be unreal. This kind of false-alarm fight-or-flight response, although less intense than the real one, can often persist for a long duration and be just as energy-draining. Can you name a few common imaginary threats that one may encounter in this modern society?

One common "imaginary threat" which many of us willingly pay money to participate comes in the form of violent, scary or high-energy entertainment — such as action and horror movies, TV shows, video games and ear-blasting music. Some say that one becomes desensitized with increased exposure to violence, but isn't it true that people watch violent movies and play war zone video games exactly for the excitement of danger and the subsequent adrenaline rush? As these types of entertainment are so commonplace, many people have been draining vital force for long hours through the many mini fight-or-flight responses without even knowing it.

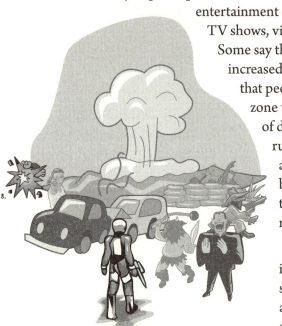

Movie scenes with armed robbery, car crashes, bomb explosions, alien invasion, blood-thirsty monsters, battle combats and gun stunts — "imaginary threats" which people call "entertainment". When done well, they are no less scary than threats in real life.

I suggest that you take an inventory of the amount of these over-stimulating entertainments which you and your family are viewing or playing, and set limits according to your daily work load and responsibilities. Most importantly, do not engage in these kinds of entertainment in the evening hours so that you can allow the body to peacefully transition into the yin (i.e. resting) state and promote good sleep. In their place, watch a relaxing or comic movie, take a warm bath or shower, read a favorite book, listen to calm music, spend some quiet time with family, or practice a chi-enhancing technique, such as chi gong (see Chapter 4).

HABIT #28:
Set limit to the amount of over-stimulating entertainments you engage in, particularly those that occur during the evening hours.

Another type of "imaginary threat", usually brought about by traumatic past events or high-stake future events, comes in the form of compulsive thinking and intense emotion.

Certainly, most life-changing events, such as death of a family member or friend, divorce with a spouse, breakup with a lover or loss of valuable property, can easily overwhelm and paralyze our mind. But we may also find ourselves overwhelmed by more trivial matters — mentally re-enacting an angry confrontation, replaying the scenario of an accident, recalling an embarrassing event at work, or repeatedly complaining about an unfair treatment. Or, if something big is looming, one may keep worrying over an uncertain future event, repeatedly projecting what-ifs and mentally playing out a range of possible outcomes, such as those of an upcoming court trial.

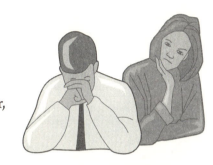
Obsessive thoughts can drain so much energy off a person that he suffers from chronic depression or anxiety attack.

In any case, these compulsive mental and emotional states can cause your brain to lose a lot of precious energy and, during the night, precious sleep — as your mind imagines the threatening situations and your body reacts with mini "fight-or-flight" responses. Worse of all, one cannot seem to stop the obsessive thoughts from resurfacing unless the brain becomes entirely drained of energy. When these types of thoughts and emotions become habitual, the body becomes trapped in an ongoing state of stress, such as chronic depression or anxiety disorder.

When one suffers from mental or emotional states so extreme that they interfere with the ability to function normally for a prolonged period of time, the problem has become too big for one individual alone to resolve — he should definitely seek professional counseling or medical help. However, if you are still capable of functioning normally and thinking rationally, there are a couple of techniques that you can use to somehow "trick" your body out of the intense mental state and back to the yin state of regeneration — meditation and physical release.

> HABIT #29:
> *Try to ease yourself out of intense mental or emotional state by using the techniques of meditation and physical release.*

The purpose of meditation is to relax the mind and the body by slowing the thought process and moving the mind into a state of awareness. There are many types of meditation, each with a special technique for quieting the mind — such as sitting upright in a quiet place and focusing the mind on the breath, an object, a mantra (word chant) or a body part. As the mind focuses, thoughts are allowed to come and go without being absorbed by the mind and, eventually, the thoughts will slow down and a state of awareness can be achieved.

In TCM, the chi-enhancing exercise called chi gong specifically combine meditation techniques with movement techniques to achieve the state of awareness (see Chapter 4). Therefore, as you practice chi gong, you can calm your mind of intense emotions and at the same time strengthen your chi flow. I strongly recommend chi gong as the preferred form of meditation.

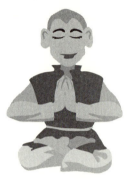

Meditation requires prior practice, but it is the best way to relax the mind and slow down unwelcome brain activities.

On the other hand, the purpose of physical release is to provide an appropriate outlet for the emotional energy and to refocus the mind away from the intense emotions. Useful physical activities can be as simple as taking a brisk walk, practicing your tennis serve or volleyball spike, or even mopping the floor. You can also channel the energy vocally by singing an upbeat song in a strong loud voice, emphasizing the rhythm of a song with your footsteps as you walk, or accompanying a song with punches to a pillow as you make the bed.

Sect. 3-5: Unnecessary heat loss

As warm-blooded animals, we humans carry a heavy burden for having to constantly maintain our body's temperature at a toasty 99°F (37°C) against the much cooler surrounding temperature of 68°F (20°C) in spring or 40°F (4°C) in winter. Obviously, body heat is constantly being lost to the environment due the drastic temperature difference — of about 60 degrees in °F (or 33 degrees in °C) in winter! In order to produce enough heat to keep up with the heat lost to the environment, our bodies, like baking ovens, have to constantly consume large amount of vital substance, even when sitting still and doing nothing.

Our homes face a similar challenge during the winter months, as the heating furnace consumes large amount of natural gas to warm up the house and much of our money get drained off for the energy bill. When the bill becomes unbearable, prudent homeowners will try to figure out ways to save energy, such as replacing windows with double-pane ones, re-caulking leaky windows, installing better insulation material in the attic, etc. As the owner of a hot oven that is your body, will you be interested in figuring out ways to save energy, too?

If so, we have good news for you: your body can achieve tremendous savings in energy without expensive remodeling or replacement as our houses do — all we need are some simple behavior modifications and the will to practice them. It turns out that the most common ways the body loses heat unnecessarily is through exposure to cold or damp conditions. So if we can reduce the impact of these conditions with the right precautions, we can save big on our energy bill — in terms of vital force. Let us examine some common situations involving cold or damp conditions and the kinds of precautions we can take.

> We have good news for you: your body can achieve tremendous savings in energy without expensive remodeling or replacement as our houses do — all we need are some simple behavior modifications and the will to practice them.

(a) Weather conditions

We become exposed to cold or damp conditions whenever we go outdoors in cold, rainy or windy weather. While chilly air or pouring rain should immediately remind us of the need to wear extra layers of clothes or to carry an umbrella, there are many occasions where poor weather conditions are not imminent and we neglect to take the necessary precautions. These are the occasions where we most likely become victims of vital force drainage.

Take, for example, the times of rapidly-fluctuating weather — most commonly during the transitions from summer to fall, fall to winter, and winter to spring. In mid October, we may leave home into the hot afternoon wearing shorts and a T-shirt but find ourselves too thin on clothes when it becomes very chilly as soon as the sun sets. In mid March, just when the temperature heats up and we begin shedding our woolly winter clothes, the weather may all of a sudden plunge back into cold, winter-like condition.

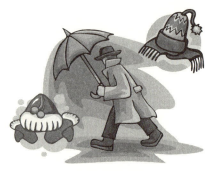

To prepare for fluctuating weather, keep on hand your jacket and hat for the wind, mittens and scarf for the cold, and your umbrella for the rain.

This is why the transitions of seasons are the times when coughing, sneezing, colds and flus are most common. While the cold and flu viruses are present throughout the year, people are most likely to be caught off guard during these times, suffer a drain of vital force, become weakened and less able to defend against the disease agents. As more bodies become the breeding grounds for the viruses, the viruses proliferate and go on to infect other immune-weakened people.

The precaution against fluctuating weather is quite simple — bring an extra jacket during these times, preferably one with a hat or hood. If you do not need to wear it, just leave it in your bag or backpack. But at the first sign of chill, put it on without delay as an insurance — if you do so now, you can always change your mind later by taking it off and lose nothing; but if you don't put it on now it will be too late if you change your mind!

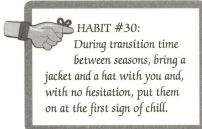

HABIT #30:
During transition time between seasons, bring a jacket and a hat with you and, with no hesitation, put them on at the first sign of chill.

Some other times, for whatever reason, people simply choose to brave the weather conditions instead of protecting themselves. On a rainy day, it is very common to see people walking in the street without any rain gear — perhaps they expect their clothes to dry quickly once they return indoors. Little do they know that wet hair, wet clothes and wet shoes can quickly draw heat away from their bodies. The lesson: don't use your body to gamble with the weather and if you ever get wet in the rain, dry your hair with a towel and change to dry clothes as soon as possible.

> **HABIT #31:**
> Prevent you hair, clothes and shoes from getting wet from rain, and if they do, dry or change them at the earliest possible instant.

Many people underestimate the effect of wind as a heat-stealer — especially through the head and neck where 30% to 50% of body heat loss occurs. In addition, when combined with cold air, the wind chill effect can drop the already-low air temperature further as detected by the skin. Thus, even in a moderately cool air temperature of 40°F, a wind speed of 10 miles per hour can effectively drop the air temperature to 34°F.

In TCM, we recognize a phenomenon called "**wind chill**" (風寒) in which parts of the body experience temperature drop due to exposure to cold wind, slowing down the flow of chi in the meridians within those areas, eventually leading to site-specific energy blockages. Such blockages can result in local symptoms like muscle aches and tendinitis, or even general symptoms like lung congestion and sinus infection when the blockages affect a wide network of meridians.

To avoid "wind chill", watch out for windy or breezy conditions, put on a hat to cover your head (a hood attached to the jacket is ideal) and avoid prolonged exposure. When indoors, watch out for situations that can possibly expose yourself to cold draft, such as when dozing off near an open window or allowing the cold air to flow directly into the room across your body.

> **HABIT #32:**
> Watch out for "wind chill": protect your head and shoulder from breezes, and stay away from cold draft near open window.

(b) Direct contact

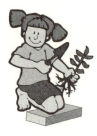

Use a foam pad as insulation from the wet ground when gardening.

We often come into direct contact with cold or damp surfaces without even knowing — picnicking on the ground or lawn, sitting on concrete, or kneeling on the ground while gardening. These are all occasions where the body can lose precious body heat. Just be mindful to place a thick insulating material between your body and the cold surface to avoid direct contact — use a rubber pad (in addition to the traditional thin blanket) while picnicking, a foam knee pad when gardening, or a foam seat cushion when attending an outdoor concert.

(c) Breathing dry or damp air

> HABIT #33:
> Avoid direct contact with cold or damp surfaces — use a layer of insulation if necessary.

In the height of winter when our homes are heated by furnaces, the very dry air they produce forces the linings of the nose, sinuses, the throat and the airways of the lungs to release moisture to counteract its drying effect. In the height of spring in humid areas where the air is cool and damp, the same linings are forced to release heat to warm the air in an attempt to preserve the body's internal temperature. In both cases, extra vital force has to be spent to replace the moisture or heat that is lost.

> HABIT #34:
> Avoid breathing in dry or damp air — use a humidifier or dehumidifier to improve the air in such conditions.

The best solution for these situations is to invest a little in technology — use a humidifier to add moisture to very dry air or a dehumidifier to reduce moisture in very damp air. These devices can also allow children to breathe more easily when sleeping.

(d) Faulty washing habits

We have to wash our hair and bodies regularly with water and every time we do so, we are exposed to wet conditions that potentially allow the rapid loss of body heat. Therefore, we have to do so intelligently to minimize the negative impact on our energy reserves. Let us carefully consider the following questions:

How often should I wash my hair? Once every three days is suitable for most people. A lot of people want to wash the hair every morning before leaving home because they cannot stand the slightest hint of oil on their hair and they want to always present the most beautiful hair at work. However, washing the hair frequently not only allows too much vital force to drain through the wet top surface, but it also over-stimulates the nerve endings in the scalp, leading to frequent headaches. Furthermore, it does take time for oil to accumulate and be noticeable on the hair — washing it daily is really not necessary.

> HABIT #35:
> *Do not wash your hair every time you shower and, when you do, blow-dry it immediately after washing.*

Should I wash my hair while taking a shower? No, the best practice is to wash your hair separately in a large sink, while fully clothed, so that you do not have to expose your wet body to cool air while taking the time to wash your hair. Similarly, you will not have to expose your scalp to a chill while your body is toweled and clothed.

What if I must shower and wash my hair at the same time? In this case, begin by making sure the bathroom air is warm, wash your body first (to minimize the time when your hair has to be wet), then wash your hair. When you are done, immediately towel dry your hair and wrap your still-wet hair in a towel, then towel dry your body, get dressed, and blow dry your hair. The goal is to minimize as much as possible the duration when your hair is wet and exposed.

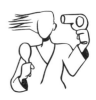

Always blow-dry your hair as soon as you finish washing — don't let wet hair come in contact with cold air.

When is the best time to wash the hair? If you are healthy with a strong reserve of vital essence, you may wash your hair at any time of the day or evening, provided that you immediately blow dry your hair. If you have health concerns and your vital essence is low, only wash your hair during the warmer times of the day.

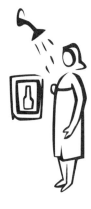

Can I leave my hair a little wet after washing? Definitely not. It always sends me a chill whenever I see men, women, boys and girls hop onto the morning bus with wet spaghetti-like hair — the most common mistake that causes body heat loss. As the water on the wet hair evaporates, it takes away heat from the scalp, forcing the body to spend large amount of energy to maintain the warmth of your head. Leaving the hair wet, even if only a little wet, greatly increases the chance of developing headaches, neck and shoulder pains, cold, flu and other respiratory problems — you should blow-dry your hair immediately after washing.

The best time to shower is at night before you go to bed.

When is the best time to shower? In the evening before bed time. Most people are accustomed to showering immediately after rising from bed as a way to wake themselves up, but moving directly from being wrapped in a warm bed to being naked in the cool bathroom runs the risk of chilling the body too rapidly, especially when one is in a hurry to work. Instead, take the shower before bed time, and you will be moving from the living room to the bathroom to the bed, without any drastic drop in air temperature. Furthermore, the act of showering can benefit your sleep by relaxing your body and mind, and preparing you for the yin state of the next eight hours.

> HABIT #36:
> Take warm shower in the evening before bed time instead of in the morning immediately after rising from bed.

Is it healthy to take hot showers? It is better to shower with warm, not hot, water. A lot of people take hot showers in the morning as a way to wake up and to get their blood rolling for the day. However, the hot water rapidly raises the body's temperature and causes the body to sweat in an attempt to cool its core temperature

— which translates to an unnecessary loss of moisture from the body. Furthermore, if the shower is taken before bed time, the hot water will increase your heart rate too much, making it more difficult for you to calm down on the bed.

(e) Highly-contrasting indoor and outdoor temperatures

With modern heating and air conditioning systems, we seem to have gained complete control over the temperature of our indoor environments — to the point where we can almost change the season. Preferring to shed their cumbersome clothes, many people turn up the heater in their homes on a cold winter day so they can eat ice cream and walk around in T-shirts and shorts. Preferring to stay sweat-free under their business clothes, many people in offices and restaurants turn up the air conditioning on a hot summer day so that they can feel the breeze of a chilly ski run.

But troubles occur when these people have to step outside of their oven-hot homes into the cold winter streets or to step from the hot summer outdoors into the chilly office buildings. At first, when the body tries to adapt to the warm temperature, the pores of the skin open, the skin sweats and the blood vessels dilate to allow for the cooling of the body. As the person quickly transits into an environment with a drastically lower temperature, the body, unable to instantly turn off its warm-weather response, experiences shock and continues to lose body heat rapidly through the open pores, wet skin and expanded blood vessels. In a very short time, the body can absorb so much dampness and cold that it falls ill — to colds and flus.

> As a person quickly transits into an environment with a drastically lower temperature, the body, unable to instantly turn off its warm-weather response, experiences shock and continues to lose body heat rapidly through the open pores, wet skin and expanded blood vessels.

> **HABIT #37:**
> *In winter, do not set the heater too high but rely on jacket and comforter to keep warm; in summer, do not set the air conditioner too low, but allow light sweating to keep cool.*

According to TCM, it is important to allow the body to experience the natural cycle of seasons and adjust to the gradual changes of weather — without the artificial confusion created by highly-contrasting indoor and outdoor temperatures. Therefore, in winter, we should set the heater at a relatively cool level of mid-60°F while relying on sweaters, woolen clothes, jackets and comforters (while sleeping) to stay warm. In summer, the air conditioning should not be set below the warm level of mid-70°F while using cool clothing and light sweating to release excess heat.

However, there are exceptions — infants, small children, elderly or persons with compromised immune systems should be kept warm at all times during winter, ideally by using a space heater, such as an electric oil-filled radiator, to warm the air of the room occupied by these vulnerable individuals.

Unfortunately, in many situations, we as guests are powerless in deciding on the settings of the heater or air conditioning. What to do when we must step out from a heated house or step into a chilly restaurant? In such cases, we will have to slow down the abrupt drop in temperature with the help of extra clothing, sometimes even when it appears to be against our own intuition.

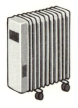

A small, mobile electric heater is ideal for keeping warm individuals who have special needs.

For example, when you are about to enter a restaurant or building with strong air conditioning, wipe off all your sweat to stop the cooling effect of evaporation and, upon entering, immediately put on an extra jacket or sweater to protect yourself from the shock of the chill — yes, even though your brain tells you it is mid-summer. Later, after your body adjusts to the cool environment and begins to feel overdressed, you can remove the extra clothing — it is the instant transition from hot to cold that is most critical.

As for stepping out into the cold outdoors, you will have to force yourself to put on enough extra layers to preserve your body heat *before* you even open the door — yes, even though you are still feeling the heat of the house furnace. Once outside, take shelter near the building for a short while to acclimatize yourself to the drastically colder condition and move out only when you feel ready. Don't overestimate your body's toughness by testing nature with your body.

> HABIT #38:
> In summer, when entering an area with strong air conditioning, immediately wipe off your sweat and put on a jacket; in winter, put on extra layers before stepping out to the cold outdoors, and take shelter to allow time for your body to adjust.

(f) Eating cold food and drinks

We have discussed in great details about the harmful effect of eating cold food and drinking cold drinks (Sect. 2-10a). I will just remind everybody that every time you eat or drink something that has been chilled with ice, the digestive tract becomes chilled to a standstill and the digestive enzymes have to take a holiday until your body heats the icy materials from 32°F (freezing point of water) to 99°F (body temperature) — a steep gap of 67 degrees in °F! This is an enormous amount of energy that should be supplied by the cooking stove or the microwave oven, not your body.

> HABIT #39:
> Do not take food or drinks that have been chilled with ice so that your body does not have to waste energy to heat them up.

X   X   X

If you have followed our discussion up to this point, you should have learned many valuable techniques and tricks for maximizing your vital substance deposited while minimizing your vital force withdrawn from your body. Once you begin to constantly achieve energy surplus every day, you are on your way to building a strong reserve of vital essence which can keep you out of energy debt for years to come. Adhere to these health habits and you will not have to worry about your fuel supply any more.

But there is more to good health than stockpiling fuel — just as happiness is more than saving money. It is time for us to focus on the fine-tuning of the body machine itself — in TCM, that means the maintenance of smooth chi flow and unobstructed meridians. That will bring us naturally to the next chapter titled "Enhancing Chi".

CHAPTER 4
ENHANCING CHI

Sect. 4-1: *The dilemma with regular exercises*

Sect. 4-2: *Non-movement-style chi gong*

Sect. 4-3: *Moving-style and martial-art-style chi gong*

Sect. 4-4: *Chi-enhancing therapies*

       (a) Acupressure

       (b) Reflexology

Sect. 4-5: *Practicing chi-enhancing techniques*

Sect. 4-1: The dilemma with regular exercises

We have discussed in Sect. 1-7 the role of chi in carrying vital substance to all parts of our bodies. In this chapter, we will focus on health habits that can strengthen the circulation of chi and my first recommendation is for you to practice a TCM-based exercise known as **chi gong** (or qigong, 氣功), specifically designed for this purpose.

In order to explain to you the concept of chi gong, I want you to first think of your favorite exercises — such as jogging through the park, swimming lapses, playing a volleyball game, shooting baskets, riding a bicycle, hiking a nature trail, playing hide-and-seek with kids, throwing a football with friends, walking your dog in the park, gardening in the backyard, vacuuming the carpet at home, etc. Now let me ask you a question: do you think exercising is good for you? I'll give you five seconds ..... OK, time's up. Let me guess: your answer is "yes", right? — I'm not surprised.

Now a slightly harder question: why do you think exercising is good for you? You can probably come up with a long list of reasons. I asked myself the same question and made the following list of benefits of exercising:

(#1) Exercising is *relaxing* — I get to do something without taxing my brain.

(#2) Exercising gives me a *change of surrounding* from the monotony of work — go out of the office to the park, the pool, the ball court, the garden, the nature trail.

(#3) Exercising lets me feel *in touch with my body* after a day of sitting still at the office pretending that my body doesn't exist.

(#4) Exercising keeps me healthy and in good shape by *stimulating metabolism, breathing and circulation* — so I can avoid heart diseases, high blood pressure, diabetes, obesity, respiratory diseases, etc.

(#5) Exercising keeps my body *slim, mobile and agile* so I don't feel clumsy and rusty when I have to walk a short distance or do physical work.

(#6) Exercising *builds strength* in my muscles and joints.

I suppose your list probably looks quite similar to this one. In making my own list, I also made a small discovery — exercising benefits a person both mentally (#1–3) and physically (#4–6).

Now, a much harder question: if exercising is so good, how come it seems so difficult to convince people to exercise? According to a 2002 poll, only 30% of women and 35% of men engaged in vigorous exercises while only "more than half" of men and women reported moderate exercise (from an article in 2004 about "benefits of exercise" on About.com by A.D.A.M., Inc.). In this era of obesity

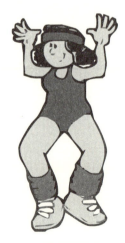

If everyone agrees that exercising is good for the body, how come so few people exercise regularly?

epidemic and fitness craze, wouldn't you expect more people to be exercising regularly? Is it the people's fault for not exercising more?

I probably would not put the blame entirely on the people themselves. It turns out that regular exercises, despite all their benefits, do have a serious drawback — they require a lot of energy and effort. That alone probably would not deter many young, able-bodied adults, but if we consider the various ages, health conditions, physical abilities, workloads and daily schedules among the wide range of people in our modern society, we may be able to understand why many people feel discouraged from exercising.

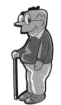
"My old bones feel cranky."

Take the elderly people, some of whom are slow to move around or even to get up, have to compromise with pains of the back, neck, arms, shoulders, knees and joints, and are prone to falling and injury. If given a choice, grandma and grandpa would rather sit at the picnic table than run around with the grandchildren. For them, exercising is not only unenticing, it is downright dangerous.

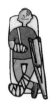
"I barely walk on clutch."

Take the sick and injured people, which include the vast majority of my patients, who may be burdened with one or more debilitating illnesses. Imagine someone whose energy level is already low from struggling with flu, indigestion, diabetes, allergy, back spasm or tendinitis — it is very difficult to ask him to do any kind of vigorous exercise.

"My head is too heavy for me to get out of bed."

Take people with obesity, who, you may think, should have totally embraced exercising as the solution to their problem. But for an overweight person, moving the hefty body continuously, with or without applied resistance, for any length of time can be a very demanding and tiring task. As exercising is viewed as a rather unpleasant experience, it is not hard to explain why these people avoid exercising, which they do not enjoy.

"A little too fast and my body will tumble."

What about our typical, healthy, 9-to-5 office workers? There certainly are many of those who exercise, or even overexercise (see Sect. 3-3). But for many more who do not exercise, the most common

"I'm so tired after a day of work."

Which of these people, do you think, are up for a workout?

reason given is "too tired and too little time". Many people are already yearning to go home after work and there are so many other more urgent things they must tend to in the four or five hours before bedtime — that exercising does not seem to be a productive way to spend the time.

It certainly does not help that most sports require that you take the time and trouble to travel to a special location, like a fitness gym (which can be expensive to join) or the tennis court (which can be dark by the time you arrive). That is why the expensive treadmill, bike machine, rowing machine or weight machine you often see on TV commercials seem so enticing when you imagine the opportunity to exercise at home. Unfortunately, if my friends and relatives are any indication, soon after the initial novelty disappears, most of these exercise machines quickly become dust collectors — with so many other things you can do or have to do at home, why waste time repeating the same silly motion on the same silly machine?

> It certainly does not help that most sports require that you take the time and trouble to travel to a special location, like a fitness gym or the tennis court.

Fitness club owners may not admit it, but it is obvious that vigorous exercise is not an attractive option for a lot of people. For some, even soft exercise that requires mild body motion seems to be mission impossible. Are there really no alternative for the elderly, the sick, the injured, the physically unfit, the tired and the busy?

Sect. 4-2: Non-movement-style chi gong

From the perspective of TCM doctors, exercising is critical for good health — and this is especially true for the sick and the injured since higher metabolism, stronger circulation and smoother respiration are exactly what the patients need. But, as we have explained earlier, if the sick and injured find it difficult to perform physical exercise, TCM doctors must find a different kind of exercise that they can do. The question is: what kind?

Therefore, thousands of years ago, TCM doctors invented a form of exercise which requires so little effort and energy that even the sick and injured can participate — but which is still capable of "strengthening chi flow". As you may recall, chi refers to the circulating energy within our bodies that carries vital substance to our organs — therefore "strengthening chi flow" is just a TCM terminology equivalent to "promoting metabolism, circulation and respiration" in our normal language. They called this form of exercise "chi gong" (which literally means "chi exercise") — specifically, the **non-movement-style chi gong** (靜功).

So how is chi gong different from regular physical exercise? Chi gong is designed with the recognition of two principles: (1) that the mind (i.e. the brain), being an inseparable part of the body, is capable of effecting physiological changes in the body, and (2) that the same kinds of physiological response brought about by external exercises involving the limbs can also be brought about by internal exercises involving the mind. Let me briefly elaborate on these two points.

In the present and in the past, we have recognized that the mind set of a person can greatly influence his recovery from diseases. My favorite example is a classical study which showed that the mere act of a friendly nurse coming to the patient's bed once in a while and pretending to make adjustment on the glucose-saline drip-delivery system — without any additional medicine — could lead to a much faster recovery, compared to those who did not have a nurse to do the same. The rational explanation was that when the patient thinks he is receiving extra care and attention, he feels more confident about his own recovery and his body somehow responds with a faster recovery.

The simple act of a nurse pretending to adjust a patient's drip-delivery system can cause measurable physiological changes in the patient — a classic example of how the mind can affect involuntary body functions.

But what exactly caused the faster recovery, if it was clearly not medicine (since the patient was not given any in this act), not the glucose-saline (since there is no change in the delivery system), and not the nurse (since the nurse did not do anything to him)? One thing we do know for certain: it is necessary for the patient to *consciously* observe the action of the nurse in order for the trick to work — implying that his *mind* must be involved. So sometimes we call it "optimism", "the will to live", "the passion for life", "the faith to get well", and other times, dismissively, we call it "superstition", "psychological effect", or even "placebo effect".

But who cares if it is just a "psychological effect", as long as it works? We are talking about the power of the mind over the functions of the body — the ability of the mind to effect physiological changes. Of course, everyone knows that the mind controls all the voluntary functions like walking, pulling, thinking, seeing, hearing and emotions — so why not involuntary functions, such as those performed by the immune system or circulatory system?

It is not a far-fetched idea at all. Just consider one possibility called the neuroendocrine connection: the neurons of the cerebrum connect with the hypothalamus (the sensory center of the brain), which controls the pituitary gland (an endocrine gland at the bottom of the brain), which secretes hormones (e.g. ACTH) that influence the adrenal cortex (in the adrenal glands), which secretes hormones (e.g. cortisol) that modulate the immune system. Similarly, the brain is connected through the spinal cord to the sympathetic nervous system, which can directly send nervous signals to the adrenal medulla (in the adrenal glands), which secretes hormones (e.g. epinephrine) that affect the circulatory and respiratory systems. The forebrain, center of the conscious mind, is, for all practical purposes, functionally connected with all parts of the body.

> In fact, the best way to use the mind to affect involuntary functions is to slow it down and allow it to be completely free of thoughts.

However, when we talk about "the mind over body", we are not talking about wishful thinking — constantly imagining a faster immune system in your mind probably will not give you anything besides anxiety. That is not how it works. In fact, quite the contrary, many different cultures, including TCM, have independently figured out that the best way to use the mind to affect involuntary functions is to slow it down and allow it to be completely free of thoughts — through some form of meditation, which brings us back to the non-movement-style chi gong.

A major component of non-movement-style chi gong is the techniques of meditation. During the practice, the person stays still either in a special sitting posture (坐功) or in a special standing pose (站樁功), the eyes remain open and the mind focuses on certain energy points on the body or on a healing natural image. As the body relaxes and the mind focuses, thoughts begin to appear but are allowed to come and go without being absorbed. Eventually, the thoughts slow down and a deep state of awareness arises.

According to TCM theory, when the mind and body reach this state, no vital force is needed to support the external activities of the body and, therefore, all the chi is able to build up and concentrate internally. Without leaking to the external world, the chi now circulates strongly through the meridians at a higher pressure than is normally possible. This strong flow of chi then results in an overall increase in metabolism, circulation and respiration — much like what happens in physical exercise. The main difference is that, instead of using external exercise of the arms and legs to induce physiological changes, non-movement-style chi gong uses internal exercise of the mind.

A pressure cooker internally creates steam of very high pressure by sealing off all the escape routes of the steam. Similarly, non-movement-style chi gong promotes chi flow internally by shutting off all external activities that allow chi to leak outward.

But, as in any real sports, don't expect instant magic — non-movement-style chi gong does require a certain amount of practicing to master. But talk to people who have practiced it for a couple of months and they can tell you that during the exercise, they can feel powerful changes in their bodies, such as warmth surging in the palms and soles, and tingling of the arms and legs. Other people find themselves burping repeatedly, or giving long sighs, or releasing gas from the bowel, or making growling noises in the stomach, or feeling warmth

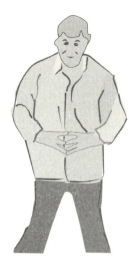

Non-movement-style chi gong involves mostly silent postures, such as this, in which a person forms a circle with his fingers near the navel while his mind focuses on the Dan Tian (丹田) acupoint.

near their sore areas, or even feeling relief from headache — all signs of various problems straightening up as the chi resumes a smooth circulation.

One of my patients, soon after practicing standing pose chi gong, reported experiencing a dull pain in the sciatica between the buttocks, which she had injured in a fall many years ago but never quite fully healed. I explained to her that this is happening because the chi flow, accelerated during chi gong, is experiencing blockage in the injured area and that she needed not be alarmed. Not surprisingly, after another day or so of chi gong practice, the dull pain disappeared — and her long-time injury had also healed.

As you can see, while non-movement-style chi gong benefits a person mentally and physically in similar ways as regular exercising does (#1–4 in my benefit list in Sect. 4-1), it also offers several advantages. Since it requires only a simple series of movements to begin and wrap up the exercise, it does not drain off precious energy from a person who is sick, injured, elderly, overweight or tired. Since it takes only 15 minutes each day and does not require any special equipment or location, it is ideal to fit into the schedule of a busy person.

Consequently, I recommend all my patients to learn and practice non-movement-style chi gong, even when they are healthy, as everyone will likely fall into one of the categories of sick, injured, elderly, out of shape, overexhausted or overstretched, at least once in a while. I suggest that they practice it for 15 minutes before bed time and right in their bedroom since the meditation exercise helps relax the mind and ease the body into peaceful sleep — a great way to relieve from insomnia, stress, overexcitement, anxiety, depression or other intense emotions.

HABIT #40:
Learn and practice non-movement-style chi gong for 15 minutes before bed time to relax the mind and body into peaceful sleep.

An important word of caution: even though side effects are rare, non-movement-style chi gong does affect the vital flow of chi and, therefore, it is very important to learn it correctly from a qualified teacher, who can comment and make corrections on your techniques in person. Don't try to save money — the cost of a chi gong class is much less than the cost of one visit to the doctor's office. The benefits gained are well worth the money.

Now what about healthy people who prefer to move around while exercising? What about the training of body agility and muscle strength (#5–6 in the benefit list in Sect. 4-1)? Well, chi gong has something to offer you. Just read on.

Sect. 4-3: Moving-style and martial-art-style chi gong

Before reading this book, many of you may already have a glimpse of chi gong from documentaries like Bill Moyer's "Healing and the Mind" (first episode: The Mystery of Chi). For many people, chi gong conjures up images of elderly people in the parks of Chinese cities, practicing soft-style, slow-motion martial art. Yet other people may associate chi gong with kung fu master brandishing spears in rapid motion, smashing stacks of wooden boards with bare hands, or effortlessly pushing back a few strong, young men.

All of these images indeed depict chi gong in action, but not in the same style as non-movement-style chi gong, which I discussed in the previous section (Sect. 4-2). It turns out there are three different levels of chi gong, depending on the level of vigor required of the performers. The non-movement-style chi gong, considered level-1 chi gong, is the least vigorous of the three.

> Tai Chi is an exquisite act of balance and concentration — if a bystander comes up and tries to push the practitioner off balance, not only will the practitioner stays on his feet, but the bystander himself will be the one who ends up tumbling on the ground.

Next, in increasing level of vigor, is the **moving-style chi gong** (level-2 chi gong), which can be very gentle to fairly demanding. For example, Tai Chi (太極), probably the gentlest form of moving-style chi gong, involves a series of slow movements centering on twenty-four to forty-eight postures derived from animals of longevity such as crane, bear, lion, dragon, etc. These pre-determined movements have been designed with the purpose of promoting the internal circulation of chi, blood and lymph, and to relieve the effects of stress.

Although Tai Chi is practiced in solo, many people enjoy practicing in synchrony with a group — and that was exactly what the slow-moving elderly Chinese people were doing in the parks. To people unfamiliar with Tai Chi, the slow motion may give the false impression that it is dull, unchallenging, trivial and non-deserving of the status of an exercise. However, Tai Chi is an exquisite act of balance and concentration — to such an extent that, if a bystander comes up and tries to push the practitioner off balance, not only will the practitioner stays on his feet, but the bystander himself will be the one who ends up tumbling on the ground!

Seeing this, the bystander will probably think that the Tai Chi practitioner must possess amazing muscles with the strength of a weightlifter and the firmness of steel. But talk with the elderly people in the park and you will be surprised to find out that they are quite normally built, often undersized, and are actually striving to keep their muscles relaxed throughout the exercise. Ask them what their "secret" is and they will tell you that the "strength" you observed comes from the redirection of the accelerated chi from within the body to the external world.

"Pushing hands" is a version of Tai Chi Chuan in which two partners take turn to push each other in a single fluid motion, emphasizing breathing, balance and relaxation.

Whether millions of elderly people are telling the truth or not, you just have to join a Tai Chi class and practice to find out. Whatever you conclude, moving-style chi gong gives you the extra benefits of improved body agility and muscle strength (benefits #5–6 in my list, in addition to benefits #1–4). However, it is important to keep in mind that moving-style chi gong is appropriate only for people who are basically healthy and not suffering from current health conditions — therefore it is best practiced for health maintenance. For the purpose of health building, choose non-movement-style chi gong.

If what appeals to you is speed, look into a fast version of moving-style chi gong, such as the well-known Tai Chi Chuan (太極拳). Tai Chi Chuan involves a series of forceful, jerky and rapid movements or postures, in coordination with the breath to activate a state of relaxation that promotes chi circulation. It can be practiced in solo or with a partner using a technique known as "pushing hands" (推手) that resembles controlled fighting or self-defense.

> HABIT #41:
> If you are in healthy condition and prefer to move around while exercising, learn and practice a version of moving-style chi gong that is suitable for you.

Even more rigorous is the **martial-art-style chi gong** (level-3 chi gong), which runs the gamut of Siu Lin Gong (少林功), Kung Fu (功夫) and many kinds of weapon manipulations. These exercises are meant for the purpose of self-defense, competition and exhibition, and are considered to be hard-style martial arts. They provide vigorous training in chi focus and control but positively require a strong healthy body and considerable time commitment for training — definitely not for the ordinary city dwellers, except the professional athletes.

As you can see, there are many styles and types of chi gong exercises for people with different health history, physical ability, lifestyle and amount of vital essence reserve. The best way to find the correct chi gong exercise for your specific situation is to consult with a TCM practitioner or chi gong instructor who is trained in the healing principles of TCM. While there are books and videos about chi gong that can serve as references, they should not replace the personal, hands-on role of an experienced chi gong instructor.

Sect. 4-4: Chi-enhancing therapies

While chi-enhancing exercise like chi gong promotes the overall circulation of chi throughout the body, there are several kinds of therapy that can be used to stimulate chi flow for specific meridians, the channels for chi flow. You are probably already familiar with acupuncture (針灸), one example of chi-enhancing therapies, in which fine needles are inserted strategically at some of the more than four hundred acupoints (or energy points, 穴位) throughout the body surface so that the chi flow through the associated meridian networks can be restored. However, acupuncture is a highly technical craft which requires the skills and knowledge of a professional acupuncturist.

For the average person, there are other kinds of chi-enhancing therapies based on the application of pressure on specific points on the body, which can be safely performed at home, perhaps with the help of an assistant. Of course, you will need to be instructed by a TCM physician as to what specific points to use and what kind of pressure to apply, but when performed properly, these self-help therapies can promote healing by enhancing your chi between your visits to the clinic. Here, I will discuss two examples of such therapies — acupressure (推拿) and reflexology (反射療法).

(a) Acupressure

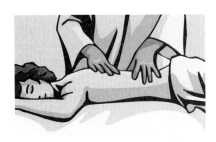

Acupressure works by stimulating acupoints along particular meridians related to a health condition.

Acupressure, also called Tui Na, in a sense, replaces the puncturing of acupuncture needles with the pressure of a thumb (or a hand, knuckle, finger, elbow or rounded wooden tool). As in acupuncture, when firm, prolonged pressure is applied on specific acupoints, the chi flow within the associated meridian networks will be stimulated. This method of acupressure is called **direct-pressure method**.

Acupressure can also be applied in a different way called **gentle-touch method**. In this method, one hand applies gentle pressure on an anchor point while another hand does the same simultaneously to a related point. This creates a bridge between the two acupoints, boosting chi flow and removing energy blocks between them.

Sometimes applying pressure to one acupoint will produce a sensation of pain in other parts of the body, called referred pain in medical terminology. This indicates that the chi flow is also blocked at those other locations. If this happens, you should apply pressure to the acupoints near the location of the referred pain so that all blockages can be released.

(b) Reflexology

Reflexology, also called zone therapy, is another chi-enhancing therapy that stimulates chi flow by applying pressure to specific points — this time, on the soles of the feet. Sometimes specific points on the palms of the hands and the ears can also be used. I am sure you must be wondering what is so special about the soles and palms, right?

According to TCM theories, a meridian (i.e. channel of chi) typically originates from a parent organ (such as the lungs or the liver), extends upward toward the head, then downward toward the hands, the torso, and the legs. Once it reaches the sole of the feet, it loops back to the organ of origin, thus forming a closed circular route for the circulation of chi. As a result, every meridian has to somehow pass through some area under the sole, making the sole a one-stop center for accessing all the meridians related to all of the body's organs.

> Each of the more than twenty meridians has to somehow pass through some area under the sole, making the sole a one-stop center for accessing all the meridians related to all of the body's organs.

Exactly which spot on the sole is associated with the meridians of which organs — that has been painstakingly mapped out by different groups of reflexologists and represented on color-coded reflexology charts. If you compare the reflexology charts from different groups, you will notice that while they more or less agree on the approximate areas and the associated organs, they do show certain degrees of variations due to subtle differences in the clinical experiences of the different groups. In fact, even today, every TCM practitioner may have his own favorite reflexology chart and continue to make modifications based on his own clinical experiences.

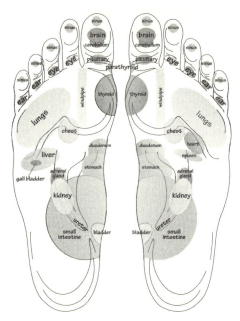

A reflexology chart showing specific areas of the soles with their related organs.

In practice, the exact positions of the reflexology points vary slightly even among individual patients and the TCM practitioner has to map out every patient's sole on the spot by testing his sensation to touch with a rounded wooden stick (called finger stick). For example, if a patient is diagnosed to be weak in kidney chi, he will feel pain when the general area of the sole corresponding to the kidneys is *gently* pressed with a finger stick. In fact, most of the time, a gentle touch with a finger stick will suffice in delivering pain, while a *firm* press on an unaffected area of the sole is quite tolerable. The TCM practitioner will then have to pinpoint the exact reflexology point by locating the point that delivers the maximum pain sensation.

In most cases, when the right reflexology point is pressed or touched, the pain is so surprisingly intense that the patient moans or even screams loudly, quickly withdrawing his foot "in protest". The patient is then instructed to continuously blow air through his mouth, which makes the pain tolerable during the several minutes of therapy. To be sure, the pain has nothing to do with any physical injury of the foot, since the patients generally feel no discomfort when walking or running — rather, it is the sensation of blocked or stagnant chi flow within the affected meridians.

> HABIT #42:
> Practice acupressure and reflexology techniques at home as instructed by your TCM practitioner in order to promote healing by enhancing chi flow.

In the clinic, during reflexology therapy, a TCM practitioner usually applies pressure on the selected acupoints with the thumb or a finger stick, firmly and in a rocking motion for a minute or two at a time. At home, with prior instructions and demonstration from the TCM practitioner, the patient can administer the same reflexology therapy with the help of an assistant. However, when an assistant is not available, other substitute tools may have to be used.

One possibility is to use a walnut with thick shell and no cracks, which can be rolled between the floor and the sole to create pressure on specific reflex points. Another possibility, although not as portable, is to use a small plastic tub filled with small river rocks to about 6 inches deep, preferably those with a combination of rounded edges and hard angles. To self-administer the therapy, simply step into the tub of rocks and alternately step from foot to foot for five to ten minutes to stimulate reflex points on the soles of the feet.

Sect. 4-5: Practicing chi-enhancing techniques

Now that you are familiar with the chi-enhancing exercises and chi-enhancing therapies available to you, the next most important question to ask is probably: when and how often should I practice these techniques?

The answer is: at least once every day. But certain times are better than others — for chi gong, the best times are (1) between waking and breakfast (e.g. 6:00 A.M. to 8:30 A.M.), (2) after work and before dinner (e.g. 5:30 P.M. to 6:30 P.M.) and (3) for non-movement-style chi gong only, one and a half hour after dinner (e.g. 9:00 P.M. to 10:30 P.M.). At these times, the digestive process either has not started for a fresh meal or has mostly slowed down for the previous meal, and thus the chi is fully available for internal circulation while the subsequent boost of energy by chi gong will help digest the next meal.

Chi-enhancing therapies, such as acupressure and reflexology, are also best practiced during the above time slots — however, wait at least twenty minutes after the end of the therapy session before eating. They can also be used throughout the day on a first-aid basis to address emerging problem of energy imbalance, such as headache, sore muscles, upset stomach or low energy. Hand reflexology for first aid has an additional advantage at the workplace or in public because it does not require special equipment or space and does not attract attention since it is practiced when fully clothed.

X   X   X

By now, you have learned the in's and out's of acquiring vital substance, conserving vital force and enhancing chi. If you put the ideas into practice, you will have done your part in saving up a strong reserve of vital essence and making sure your chi flows strongly and smoothly. With these in place, you are finally ready to harvest the healing power of your own body to achieve good health.

There is just one more step — you have to give your self-healing power the chance to work on your body. How? What do you have to do? Ironically, you do this is by taking the time to not do anything, which will be the topic of next chapter.

CHAPTER 5
PROMOTING SELF-HEALING

Sect. 5-1: *Your other job starts at 10:30 P.M.*

Sect. 5-2: *The meridian clock of self-regeneration*

Sect. 5-3: *Why the liver holds the key to all diseases*

      (a) On digestive system

      (b) On excretory system

      (c) On nervous system

      (d) On endocrine and reproductive systems

      (e) On immune system

      (f) On circulatory system

Sect. 5-4: *Liver and gall bladder have the most hazardous job of all*

      (a) Extreme blood

      (b) Food-borne pathogens

      (c) Natural and artificial toxins

      (d) Reactive oxygen species

      (e) Gallstones

      (f) Blood congestion

      (g) Emotional stress

Sect. 5-5: *The TCM strategy for a healthy liver*

Sect. 5-6: *Promoting good-quality sleep*

Sect. 5-7: *Recharging during the day*

      (a) Regular breaks

      (b) Lunch break

      (c) Overtime work

Sect. 5-8: Recharging throughout the year
    (a) Winter dormancy
    (b) Vacations
    (c) Hobbies

Sect. 5-1: Your other job starts at 10:30 P.M.

Suppose you are the CEO of an international airline. Of course, your job is to transport people from place to place with your airplanes and, in the process, make a profit with ticket sales. But you have another equally important job, although invisible to the public and occurring in the background when the airplanes are idle, of repairing and maintaining them to their best conditions. You cannot afford any mechanical malfunction in the air or even on the ground because that will be disastrous to your company's productivity.

This is the perfect analogy for all of us, productive adults in a modern society. You are the CEO of yourself, making money by providing services to your boss or customers — that is your first job. But, just as importantly, you are responsible for the other job of repairing and maintaining your means of production — in this case, your own body machine, which you rely on to remain productive. The only difference here is that, while you can hire mechanics to maintain your airplanes, you yourself have to maintain your body — no one else can do it for you, no matter how much money you have and how many people you hire — because it is your own body.

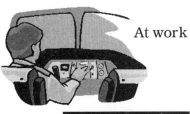
At work

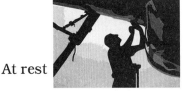
At rest

There are two phases in the daily life of an airplane: at work and at rest. No doubt, you will agree that what happens at rest is equally important as what happens at work.

True, you can hire doctors, nurses or lab technicians, but they can only give advice. True, you can buy medicine, injections, therapies or surgeries, but they can only intervene when your body has already malfunctioned — when you are already in the disastrous state of disease. To prevent diseases— that is, to prevent your body from malfunctioning — you are the only one who can repair the worn-out muscle fibers and tendons, clean off toxins and infectious agents, and regenerate retired blood cells, skin cells, intestinal cells, etc. (previously explained in Sect. 1-8).

So you really have two jobs — a day job called *work* and a night job called *rest* (when the self-healing process occurs). The two are interdependent — neglecting your day job, you are out of food and become hungry on bed; neglecting your night job, you are out of health and become sick on the job. Unfortunately, while the day job takes most of our attention, the night job is invisible, in the background, and easy to be neglected by busy, hard-working people, like you and me.

This chapter is about that often-neglected night job, the success of which ultimately determines the status of your health (see Sect. 1-9). If you have read this book up to this point, you should have understood that the purpose of all the previous chapters was simply to prepare you for this mysterious night job of self-healing. In fact, out of the three requirements for successful self-healing, you have already accomplished two — an abundant surplus of *vital essence*, and a strong *chi circulation* to supply the organs.

There is just one more requirement for the magic power of self healing — *time for rest*. That means you have to take the time to slow down from work and enter the yin state of rest so that your body can channel all its energy inward to perform self-healing.

"10:30 P.M." is the secret! Go to bed at this time and your self-healing program will have the best chance to succeed. Read on to find out why.

But not just any time of the day, as all times are not equal. TCM dictates that your night job of rest lasts 7 to 8 hours and you have to report to work at 10:30 P.M., which is the time you should go to bed. Why 10:30 P.M.? Why can't we wait till later? Well, in order to answer that question, I have to first explain a concept in TCM called the meridian clock (子午流注).

Sect. 5-2: The meridian clock of self-regeneration

For many centuries, TCM doctors have observed that symptoms related to a certain organ are most likely to occur at a certain time period of the day. For example, chills, hot flashes, nose congestion, coughing and asthma, which are symptoms related to the lungs (considered to be the regulator of body temperature according to TCM classification), are most likely to occur between the hours of 3 A.M. to 5 A.M. Similarly, symptoms related to the bowel (or large intestine) are most likely to occur between the hours of 5 A.M. to 7 A.M.

In order to explain these observations, TCM theorizes that, at any one time, the body focuses a strong current of chi internally towards one of twelve organs through its corresponding meridian network. Once every two hours, the chi current is redirected to a different meridian network according to a strict daily schedule so that each of the twelve organs receive the fortified chi current for two hours every day.

According to a strict daily schedule, each of the twelve organs receive the fortified chi current for two hours every day.

Thus, an interesting phenomenon occurs: if a certain organ of a person suffers from blockage of chi flow, he will experience symptoms of that organ when the extra-strength chi current tries to force its way through the blocked meridian. Remember that in TCM, diseases of an organ are interpreted as the effect of chi blockage in the corresponding meridian network (see Sect. 1-7)? Therefore, since lung-related symptoms are most severe during the period between 3 A.M. to 5 A.M., this must be the time when the fortified chi current is directed through the lung-related meridian network.

In this manner, TCM doctors long ago had clinically deduced the daily schedule of the fortified chi current — simply by observing what organs are most vulnerable at what time of a day. The resulting schedule, called the "**meridian clock**" (子午流注), looks something like this:

3 A.M. to 5 A.M. — Lungs
5 A.M. to 7 A.M. — Large intestine
7 A.M. to 9 A.M. — Stomach
9 A.M. to 11 A.M. — Spleen
11 A.M. to 1 P.M. — Heart
1 P.M. to 3 P.M. — Small intestine
3 P.M. to 5 P.M. — Bladder
5 P.M. to 7 P.M. — Kidney
7 P.M. to 9 P.M. — Pericardium
9 P.M. to 11 P.M. — Triple warmer (三焦)
11 P.M. to 1 A.M. — Gall bladder
1 A.M. to 3 A.M. — Liver

Now that we understand how the fortified chi current moves around our body in two-hour increments, you may wonder what we can do with this knowledge. Can we possibly take advantage of the fortified chi current for improving our health? Of course, the answer is yes — or else we would not be talking about it. But to understand how, you have to know something about the liver and gall bladder.

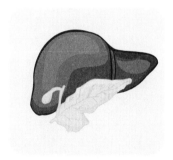

Believe it or not, having a healthy liver is the best way to prevent a large number of diseases.

Sect. 5-3: Why the liver holds the key to all diseases

There is an old saying in TCM that all diseases have their origins in the liver, from the day a person is born to the day he dies — an acknowledgment of the central role which the liver plays in a person's health. Like all proverbs, it carries a certain degree of exaggeration but also a certain degree of truth and wisdom. Just think about this: while jaundice (yellowing of the skin) is one of the most common health conditions in newborns, gall bladder stone is the cause of one of the most common surgical operations among adults in the U.S. and type II diabetes is one of the leading causes of death in the U.S. All three diseases occur because of liver malfunction.

The liver has long been recognized as the most versatile organ in our body — so much so that, unlike the heart, kidney and lungs, there is no artificial replacement for the liver. In fact, every day, the normal liver must perform such a huge variety (500+) of functions that if it becomes inefficient for even a short time, problems are bound to occur somewhere in some organ system of the body. In short, every organ in the body directly or indirectly relies on the liver. In a moment, you will appreciate the enormous influence of the liver on all parts of the body.

(a) On digestive system

The liver is commonly regarded as an accessory gland of the digestive system, as we have already discussed how the liver produces bile salts, necessary for the digestion of lipids and the lubrication of the intestines (see Sect. 2-4). In addition, it acts as the dam that holds back the flood of nutrients rushing into the blood circulation from the digestive tract after a meal — or else we will suffer from diabetes when blood sugar surges to a dangerously high level. In fact, the liver cells are responsible for maintaining a balanced level of sugar, lipids, amino acids, minerals and vitamins, by storing or breaking them down when there are too much and synthesizing them when there are too little.

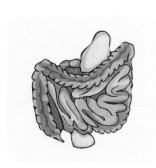

The liver produces bile for fat digestion and regulates the level of nutrients into blood.

(b) On excretory system

Besides its involvement with nutrients, the liver's most important job has to be the destruction and elimination of toxic chemicals in blood. When blood enters the liver, it is led into an extensive network of capillaries called hepatic sinusoids, which are tiny blood vessels full of holes so that the liquid portion of the blood (plasma) can readily leak out of the sinusoids to form lymph. Standing guard immediately outside the sinusoids are the liver cells, which constantly sample the lymph fluid and immediately pick up and destroy any toxic chemicals it can find.

What kinds of toxic chemicals? The most important one is ammonia, which is constantly produced whenever amino acids (from proteins) are converted to carbohydrates or fats, as well as by bacteria residing in the intestine. Ammonia, the same pungent chemical sold as toilet cleaner in supermarket, is extremely toxic and the

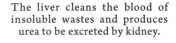

The liver cleans the blood of insoluble wastes and produces urea to be excreted by kidney.

liver cells must quickly catch it from the blood and convert it into urea, which is much less toxic, to be excreted through the kidney in urine. Thus, the liver, like the kidneys, is a major organ of the excretory system.

Another example of toxic chemical is bilirubin, which is the substance that gives the yellow color in urine and in feces (after some chemical modifications). When old red blood cells die (and about 3 million of them die every second!), the red pigment inside (hemoglobin) spills out and breaks down into bilirubin. Bilirubin is toxic and, within hours of its appearance in blood, the liver cells will absorb it, chemically process it, and transport it out of the liver through a special canal system (bile canaliculi) into the bile duct, and into the gall bladder to become part of bile, to be discarded through the intestine together with feces. If the liver cells are unable to efficiently clean up the toxic bilirubin from blood, it stays in the blood and the person's skin becomes tainted with a greenish yellow color — the symptom of jaundice.

In fact, the bile is a major excretory route by which the body get rid of large (in molecular size) and water-*insoluble* wastes, just as urine is the major exit route for water-*soluble* wastes. Besides bilirubin, many other organic wastes, including cholesterol, steroid hormones, many types of drugs and dyes, are also eliminated through the bile and gall bladder system. The implication is enormous — without the prompt action of healthy liver cells, all kinds of organic wastes will accumulate in our bodies.

(c) On nervous system

As toxic chemicals begin to accumulate in blood and body fluid when the liver fails to function, the most immediately-affected organ system is probably the nervous system because delicate nerve cells are particularly sensitive to toxins. For example, the organs most negatively affected by alcoholism are the liver and the brain. In fact, it has long been recognized by TCM that one of the first signs of liver failure occurs with the eyes, a major organ of the nervous system, which become very prone to fatigue, such as from watching TV and reading books.

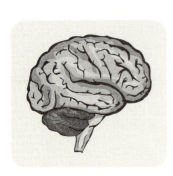

Whenever the liver has problem keeping up with the burden of detoxification, the brain is the first organ to show symptoms.

Liver failure may also contributes to terminal brain diseases such as Alzheimer's Disease and Parkinson's Disease. These diseases are believed to be caused by misfolded proteins (called amyloid-beta protein) that tangle up into toxic plaques within brain cells. Normally, the circulating blood acts as a sink for these proteins to escape the brain and be delivered to the liver cells for destruction. But if the weakened liver fails to clear the amyloid-beta protein off the blood, it accumulates in the brain and end up in tangles, killing the brain cells with the passage of time.

(d) On endocrine and reproductive systems

All the hormones produced by endocrine glands are meant to stay in the body only for a short period of time and the liver plays an important role in regulating the effects of hormones by adjusting the speed of clearance from the bloodstream. This is best illustrated with the menstrual cycle of women, in which the levels of hormones such as estrogen and progesterone have to go up and come down in a precise schedule. When the weakened liver fails to clear off these hormones in a timely manner, the timing of the responses of uterus and ovary become chaotic, resulting in irregular menstruation, lack of menstrual flow, excessive menstrual flow, severe premenstrual syndrome and even infertility.

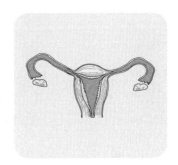

When the liver fails to properly regulate the levels of reproductive hormones, the reproductive system suffers from dysfunction and abnormal growth.

Estrogen and testosterone are also highly mitogenic to many cell types, meaning that cells are stimulated to divide and multiply by these hormones. This is particularly true for organs related to the reproductive system, such as uterus, ovary, breasts and prostate gland. As a result, when the clearance of estrogen or testosterone by the liver is inefficient, these hormones accumulate in body tissues and may lead to abnormal tissue growth such as endometriosis, uterine fibroid, ovarian cyst, breast tumor and enlarged prostate.

(e) On immune system

Ingested food is laden with all kinds of foreign agents that can potentially cause diseases. In fact, one can routinely obtain bacterial colonies simply by culturing a sample of the portal blood which enters the liver from the intestine. The liver, as a first-line defense against these invaders, has a large number of specialized white blood cells (called Kupffer cells) patrolling the hepatic sinusoids, constantly grabbing and

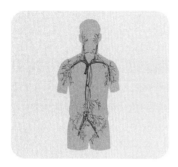

Along with lymph nodes and spleen, the liver is one of the major centers for the sampling of

engulfing these foreign bodies from the blood. As a result, by the time the blood leaves the liver, more than 99% of the bacteria has been removed — a testament to the high efficiency of the liver as a blood cleansing filter.

As the bacteria and viruses are digested by the Kupffer cells, the resulting bits and pieces are presented to helper T-lymphocytes (another type of white blood cells), which in turn can mobilize the immune system to produce the appropriate antibodies to fight similar bacteria or viruses. Obviously, without the vigilance of the Kupffer cells in the liver, the response of the immune system to infectious diseases will be inefficient and much delayed.

(f) On circulatory system

The performance of the liver directly affects the function of the circulatory system due to the sheer volume of blood it processes each minute — at resting, approximately 1.4 to 1.5 liter of blood flows into and out of the liver. Such amount is astounding because, while the liver only accounts for 2% of the body weight, the blood input of the liver alone accounts for 30% of blood pumped out of the heart in one minute. Obviously, if the heart is to continue to deliver blood normally to all parts of the body, the liver must be able return 1.4 to 1.5 liter of the blood back to the heart every minute — any congestion of blood flow within the liver can cause serious problem to the heart.

On the other hand, if blood flow ever becomes congested in the right atrium of the heart, the liver can act as an emergency reservoir to hold an additional 0.5 to 1.0 liter of blood as the back pressure causes the liver to expand. Thus, the liver acts as an effective buffer, like a sponge, capable of storing up excess blood (when the blood volume increases) and of supplying extra blood back to the peripheral circulation (when the blood volume decreases, such as during severe bleeding).

Speaking of blood, the liver is responsible for producing 90% of all the proteins found in the plasma (the remaining 10% being mostly antibodies, called immunoglobulins, produced by plasma cells of the immune system). These proteins include a whole series of clotting proteins, responsible for sealing up wounds of damaged blood vessels, or else excessive bleeding or hemophilia is the result. Another important plasma protein produced by the liver is albumin, which serves to provide the necessary osmolarity (i.e. concentration of dissolved substances) in blood so that the water content of blood can be maintained without being lost to tissue fluid. Edema or tissue swelling is the result when albumin is not sufficiently produced by the liver cells.

As we have mentioned earlier, red blood cells (erythrocytes) in blood has a fairly short life span and when they start falling apart, the Kupffer cells in the liver, along with macrophages (the counterpart of Kupffer cells) in the spleen, are responsible for dismantling them and recycling their hemoglobin content. The most precious part of hemoglobin is the iron, which is passed to liver cells to be stored in a protein-bound form called ferritin — which later releases the iron back to the blood when the blood iron level is low. Just imagine what will happen if the liver cells fail to recycle and store the precious iron — the loss of iron will become too large to be offset by dietary iron. Without enough iron, we cannot make enough hemoglobin and anemia will be the result.

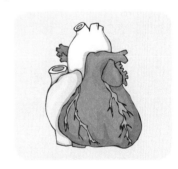

The liver maintains many components of the blood, including blood proteins, blood cholesterol and red blood cells.

Atherosclerosis, which is the main cause of heart attack and stroke, is caused by the buildup of cholesterol plaques along the wall of arteries, partially clogging these major conduits and inappropriately triggering internal blood clotting (thrombosis). In a healthy person eating a normal diet, the liver is responsible for synthesizing and converting cholesterol into bile salts to be used in bile for lipid digestion and destroying any excess circulating cholesterol bound to lipoproteins. As you can imagine, there should not be any extra cholesterol left to form atherosclerotic plagues — unless, you guess it, the liver fails to do its job.

By now, I hope you can fully appreciate the remarkable contributions of our largest internal organ, the liver. To the honor of the liver, TCM often claims that, if all the organs in our body must work together as an army, then the liver must be the general. Yet, much of the functions it performs lie in the background and are largely unnoticed — until something goes wrong somewhere in some organ far, far away.

Sect. 5-4: Liver and gall bladder have the most hazardous job of all

Precisely because of the kind of jobs they perform, liver cells are constantly exposed to insults and injuries while on the line of duty. The heroism of the liver can only be appreciated when we understand all the hazards it face on a daily basis.

(a) Extreme blood

Liver cells routinely handle hazardous materials that easily kill most other cells types. As the flood gate between the digestive system and the systemic blood circulation, the liver has to receive blood containing toxic levels of sugar, amino acids, lipids, vitamins and minerals — in fact, the highest concentrations anywhere in the body. If blood that rich in nutrients ever reaches the brain, it will promptly shock a person into unconsciousness.

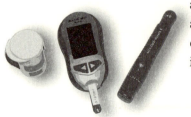

Anyone who self-monitors for diabetes has first-hand experience with the dramatic rise of the sugar level in blood after every meal.

(b) Food-borne pathogens

As nutrients take a ride through the portal vein into the liver, so do any bacteria and viruses that enter the intestine via food, having survived the stomach acid. Some of these food-borne pathogens can be lethal and their names have become familiar medical terms — *Clostridium botulinum, E. coli* (0157:H7 strain), *Giardia, Listeria, Salmonella, Staphylococcus, Shigella, Vibrio, Yersinia,* Hepatitus A virus, etc. Needless to say, the Kupffer cells in liver have to face the challenge of a large variety of microorganisms every day and the liver is under constant threat of infection and inflammation.

(c) Natural and artificial toxins

As a major center for detoxification, the liver cells have to collect and concentrate all kinds of toxins within themselves. Not only are there the natural toxins produced by the cells of our own bodies, such as ammonia and bilirubin, but also those that we somehow allow to enter our bodies, such as alcohol, food additives, preservatives, dietary supplements, environmental toxins, insecticides, heavy metals, dyes, pain killers, birth control pills, recreational drugs and prescription drugs. When these toxic chemicals overwhelm the capacity of the liver, the liver cells will die in large quantity, resulting in liver cirrhosis.

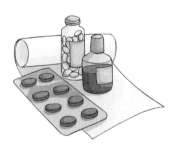

All drugs, good or bad ones, are toxins of varying degrees, which add to the long list of hazardous materials that overburden our liver cells.

(d) Reactive oxygen species

In order to destroy the large variety of organic toxins, the liver cells utilize a biochemical process called drug metabolism pathway in which a battery of highly reactive chemicals, such as peroxides, superoxide anions and other reactive oxygen species (ROS) are produced to hit the toxins. However, this brute-force method of toxic cleanup does present a catch-22 to our liver cells: these ROS are also highly reactive with vital cell components, such as DNA and plasma membranes, causing damages and premature aging to the liver cells. In fact, the liver cells have to quickly mop up any unreacted ROS with antioxidants, but, inevitably, some runaway ROS molecules do escape and cause damages to the liver cells.

(e) Gallstones

The disposal of organic wastes through bile is another tricky issue that the liver has to contend with, since bile is a water-based solution while most organic wastes, such as cholesterol, are poorly soluble in water. This situation is very similar to what many people face when washing dishes as they pour oil and grease down the kitchen sink and flush them with water — a little too much grease and the drainage becomes clogged. Our bodies face the same problem and, in order to prevent organic wastes from clogging the bile duct and gall bladder, a proper flow rate of bile and a delicate balance of the bile composition must be carefully maintained to keep the organic wastes in solution.

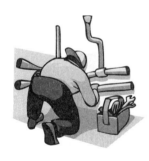

You call the plumber when your water pipes are clogged with greasy deposit. What if your bile duct is clogged with precipitation of organic wastes?

Unfortunately, things do sometimes go wrong — when the flow of bile is disrupted or when the composition of the bile is slightly off balance, cholesterol or calcium salt precipitates and crystallizes into insoluble clumps within the bile duct or gall bladder. These clumps are the dreaded gallstones which, if relatively small, will slow down the flow of bile and decrease the excretory efficiency of liver. If the gallstones are large, however, the bile ducts may be blocked, causing the toxic bile to back up into the liver, poisoning the liver cells, and triggering acute inflammation and intense pain that require emergency care. In fact, in the U.S., 25 million people suffer from gallstones at any particular time and one million new cases emerge every year. No wonder the removal of gall bladder is one of the most common surgical operations in the U. S. — 500,000 such operations are performed each year.

(f) Blood congestion

Yet more dangers are lurking around. Scientists were astounded when they first measured the pressure of blood in the portal vein entering the liver (averaging 9 mm Hg) and that in the hepatic vein leaving the liver (averaging 0 mm Hg) — how could such a small difference (9 mm Hg) in pressure push through such a large volume (1.4 liter) of blood every minute? It turns out that the hepatic sinusoids are so exquisitely designed in branching angles and surface properties that it presents very, very little resistance to blood flow — the blood simply glides swiftly and effortlessly through the slippery sinusoids.

For this exact reason, any abnormal resistance, however slight, can greatly interrupt the flow of blood through the sinusoids and cause disasters to liver functions. Such an interruption commonly occurs in liver cirrhosis when the death of injured liver cells outpaces the regeneration of new liver cells, resulting in the replacement of dead cells with fibrous connective tissues. Unlike live liver cells, however, fibrous tissues often contract around the sinusoids, partially closing them up and creating blood congestions — the liver's version of traffic jam. When the blood flow is slowed, the cleansing operation by the liver comes to a standstill and toxic wastes accumulate throughout the body.

The effect of constricted sinusoids on liver blood flow is similar to that of "merging lanes" on highway traffic.

(g) Emotional stress

It has long been recognized in TCM that the liver is particularly vulnerable to long-term stress (e.g. anxiety over performance evaluations) and extreme emotions (e.g. anger, frustration). In TCM language, stress and extreme emotions ignite "**liver fire**" (肝火), a kind of overheating of the liver. "Liver fire", in turn, causes "**liver stagnation**" (肝屈), referring to a general slow down of liver chi and, consequently, liver functions, which then causes a whole category of health conditions including insomnia, tired eyes, constant thirst, indigestion, constipation, over-reaction, irritability and hot temper. As you can see, "liver stagnation" can cause extreme emotion, which then causes more "liver fire", which, in return, causes more "liver stagnation" — and the cycle repeats.

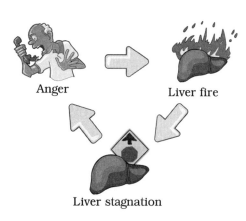

Strong emotion (e.g. anger) can cause ever-increasing slow-down of liver functions (liver stagnation) via a positive feedback loop.

This issue is particularly pertinent to modern life, which is characterized by intense competitions, high expectations, fast production cycles and lack of job security. Not surprisingly, modern science has also been studying the physiological effects due to stress and is beginning to accumulate evidence that supports a relationship between stress and the decline of liver functions.

In terms of physiology, we all know that, as part of our fight-or-flight responses, our blood pressure shoots up when we are under stress or extreme emotions. It turns out that one of the major hormones produced during stress is glucocorticoids (from the adrenal gland), a potent vasoconstrictor which down-regulates the signal (nitric oxide) that tells smooth muscle to relax. Needless to say, the most affected blood vessels are those with thick layers of smooth muscle, such as the hepatic vein which carries blood from the liver to the heart and is traveled by 30% of the total blood volume of our bodies every minute (see Sect. 5-3f, On circulating system).

When the hepatic vein constricts during a period of stress, the back pressure pushes into the liver and the liver expands to accommodate the sudden pool of blood delayed by the traffic jam. If this is a short-term stress, such as when we have to run for a bus about to depart, the congestion will be relieved as soon as the stress disappears. However, if the stress is long-term, such as when we have to beat a project deadline in 7 days or when a loved one in the family dies, the liver congestion will become long-lasting and its negative effects will become far-reaching to our health.

Although multiple factors are at play, the congestion of liver blood flow probably explains why gallstones are more likely to occur in people who are under the stress of heavy workload and why so many people go into a long period of poor health after the death of family members. The important point here is to understand that stress and emotions must not be dismissed as mere psychological issues because they are actually physiological issues that greatly affect the internal organs, particularly the liver, which, in turn, affects the health of the whole body.

> The congestion of liver blood flow probably explains why gallstones are more likely to occur in people who are under the stress of heavy workload and why so many people go into a long period of poor health after the death of family members.

Sect. 5-5: The TCM strategy for a healthy liver

Let us summarize what we have said about the liver so far. We have learned that the liver is a highly versatile organ that performs a wide range of critical tasks in the background, quietly keeping the internal chemistry of the body in check and supporting the normal functions of many organ systems. Unless we fully understand this concept, we risk hopelessly focusing on the organs of symptoms, such as the eyes with blurry vision, the arteries with cholesterol deposits, the head with hot temper, the legs with edema, or the uterus with fibroid growth — without realizing what needs to be cured are not those organs but the liver.

We have also learned that because of the nature of its jobs, the liver is constantly exposed to injuries from multiple sources: concentrated nutrients, toxins, reactive oxygen species, pathogens, gallstones, high blood pressure, long-term stress and extreme emotions. In our modern society, these sources of injuries are more common than ever — consumption of rich, processed foods and dietary supplements, over-medication (such as pain killers and antibiotics), use of mood-altering drugs and alcohol, exposure to toxins from the polluted environment, and leading a lifestyle with stressful work schedule, punctuated with over-stimulating entertainment. "Ambush from ten sides" (十面埋伏) is indeed waiting for our livers.

Fortunately, the liver is not totally defenseless. Our liver is equipped to take heavy casualties for it is the only internal organ that has the remarkable ability to regenerate — the ability to generate fresh new cells and to rebuild any damaged part. In fact, the liver's ability to regenerate is so amazing that even if three-fourths of the liver is removed, the remaining one-fourth is sufficient to grow back the entire organ.

However, even with its wonderful regenerative power, the liver has its limits — it can become overwhelmed by excessive toxins and is no match against the effects of modern-day long-term stress. The question is: what strategy do we have to counter these threats? Is there additional help we can recruit to tilt the balance in favor of our liver and gall bladder?

Let me tell you more about flying an airplane. If you have ever traveled to Asia on a jumbo 747, you may have noticed that a direct flight westward from San Francisco to Hong Kong takes almost 15 hours

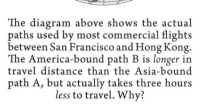

The diagram above shows the actual paths used by most commercial flights between San Francisco and Hong Kong. The America-bound path B is *longer* in travel distance than the Asia-bound path A, but actually takes three hours *less* to travel. Why?

but the reverse trip eastward, although longer in travel distance, actually takes only 12 hours. Do you know why?

Back in World War II, American fighter jet pilots discovered the "jet stream" — a fast westerly wind that blows eastward from Asia to North America over the Pacific Ocean at high altitude (about 36000 feet). Today, not surprisingly, commercial airliners flying eastward across the Pacific Ocean routinely "ride" the jet stream, which cuts the flight time by 3 hours, saving plenty of fuel and offering extra comfort for North-Amercia-bound passengers.

Why are we talking about the jet stream? Because the liver has a "jet stream" of its own — the fortified chi that is directed to the liver between 1 A.M. and 3 A.M. every night (recall from Sect. 5-2). If the liver is allowed to utilize this extra energy for its nightly self-healing, the job can be accomplished with the least amount of effort and with the highest efficiency. So how do you "allow" your liver to ride the fortified chi? You simply have to place your body in the resting yin state during this time period — that means deep sleep.

But there is more to it — since the liver and the gall bladder work as a team, any toxic wastes captured by the liver are passed to the gall bladder in high concentration (in the form of bile) for storage and elimination. That means: (1) the gall bladder is exposed to the same kinds of chemical injury faced by the liver, and (2) any problem with the gall bladder will interrupt the flow of bile and directly affect the health of the liver. Thus, if we are to protect the health of the liver, we must begin by protecting the health of the gall bladder.

Our best strategy, therefore, is to give the gall bladder the same "jet stream" advantage so that it can efficiently heal itself from chemical injuries, too. That, according to the meridian clock, occurs between 11 P.M. and 1 A.M. and so we have to be in deep sleep by 11 P.M. That, ladies

> HABIT #43:
> Go to bed promptly at 10:30 P.M. every night so that you will be in deep sleep by 11:00 P.M. for the gall bladder fortified chi (11 P.M. - 1 A.M.) and liver fortified chi (1 A.M. - 3A.M.).

and gentlemen, is why your "other night job" starts at 10:30 P.M. — the time to go to bed for the long night's sleep.

Thus, all the discussions about the meridian clock and the liver could be summarized in a single sentence: "Go to bed at 10:30 P.M. and sleep for eight hours every night." You may wonder why I didn't just say so, but when I just told my sleep-deprived patients to follow this simple instruction, a week later, they often reported that they had not done so because, as they explained, either they had too much work to do or they didn't feel the need to go to sleep that early. I then had to go through the stories of the meridian clock and the central role of the liver as related to their individual illnesses, making sure they understood that the direction to sleep at 10:30 P.M. was really not an option, but part of the prescribed "medication".

> HABIT #44:
> Give yourself 8 hours of sleep so your body has sufficient time to fully self-regenerate.

It was not until then that they became motivated to drop their work to go catch their nightly "jet stream". As they began to see their health improve, they also began placing a higher priority on sleeping promptly and treating it as seriously as their day job. As I have been telling them, you are going to *work* when you go to *sleep* — in fact, you start working on your body only *after* you go to sleep.

Sect. 5-6: Promoting good-quality sleep

> HABIT #45:
> Go to bed at the same time every night so that your body can anticipate the coming yin state and naturally fall asleep.

For most people, mustering the courage and determination to stop working and go to sleep at 10:30 P.M. is the most difficult obstacle. But once you overcome this first step, there are plenty of tips that can help you enjoy a good night's sleep and achieve maximum self-healing.

Try, as often as possible, to go to bed at the same time every night so that your body's circadian rhythm can anticipate the coming yin state and naturally tell your mind to fall asleep at the right time. Avoid casually break the routine or you will find yourself wasting an hour or more staring blankly at the ceiling when lying on bed. If there is unfinished work to do, you will take care of it when you wake up early in the morning.

> HABIT #46:
> Allow two to three hours between the end of dinner and the beginning of bedtime so your digestive system can rest when you sleep.

Give yourself two to three hours after dinner before going to bed — you want to get the heavy-lifting part of digestion out of the way in order to devote all your energy during sleep to self-healing. Furthermore, refrain from eating or drinking any significant amount after dinner or else your stomach will never finish its job in time. If you feel the need to eat before bedtime due to hunger, which should not be the case, that is a sign that the quantity of your meal was not adequate to supply your body with nutrients and fluids.

Do not over-stimulate yourself in the hours preceding bedtime in order to prepare your body and mind to enter a state of deep relaxation. Definitely do not engage in any vigorous exercise that sends your heart pounding and your blood rushing — that means no evening visit to the gym and no jogging in the dimly-lit streets. In addition, do not stir up your emotion with violent, scary or high-energy TV programs, movies, video games or music.

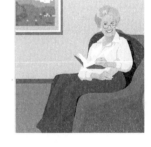

Leisure reading before bedtime is a great way to prepare for peaceful sleep.

Instead, do something that slows down your pace, such as listening to calm music, spending quiet time with family members, or reading a book at a quiet corner. Other relaxing activities I have previously recommended include taking a relaxing shower, practicing chi gong meditation for 15 minutes, or using reflexology techniques to release

> HABIT #47:
> Prepare yourself to sleep by doing something that slows down your pace and, of course, do not over-stimulate yourself with vigorous exercise or high-power entertainment.

> HABIT #48:
> Make you sleeping environment comfortable — do not overheat or overcool the bedroom and do not allow cold draft near your bed.

any energy blocks acquired during the day. Chi gong, in particular, can simultaneously calm your body for sleep and improve chi flow for the upcoming self-healing session during sleep.

Finally, you want to make your sleeping environment comfortable. During a cold night, make sure the bedroom is not overheated and, during a warm night, open a window just enough to let in fresh air and to provide air circulation. If you are to open a window, be sure that it is not near the bed and does not let in a draft over the bed — or else, it may cause the body to chill, negatively affecting chi flow when it is needed most for self-healing.

When the body is in the habit of acquiring the right food and regular rest, sleep should come within five to ten minutes of going to bed and continue uninterrupted for eight hours. There should be few dreams and the dreams that do occur should be of a pleasant nature — frequent restless and anxious dreams are indicative of energetic imbalance. When dawn arrives, if your body wakes quickly and is ready to start the day with energy, you know you have just accomplished a night of good, recharging sleep.

Sect. 5-7: Recharging during the day

So far, we have focused on the major rest period of the day, which we call sleep. But, in fact, the same principle of "wear and tear during work and self-repair during rest" applies throughout the day. It is essential that we take regular breaks throughout our work schedule to allow our engines to cool down and our batteries to recharge from time to time.

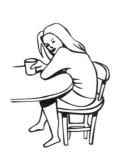

Sleeping is not the only way to rest. Short breaks work well for the mind to relax, too.

(a) Regular breaks

My rule of thumb is to take a ten-to-fifteen-minute break for every two hours of concentrated work (also discussed in Sect. 3-2). As a brief period of recharging, a good break should (1) offer you a change of activity and focus, and (2) temporarily shift your body from a responsibility-driven yang state to a self-focused yin state. For example, if your job involves sitting at a desk in front of a computer, the break should include physical activity, such as getting up and stretching the body, or walking around in the building; if your job involves physical labor, the break needs to include physical rest such as sitting down, reading a few pages of a magazine, or chatting about non-work topics with coworkers.

> HABIT #25: (repeat)
> Take a 10-to-15-minute break for every two hours of work in order to avoid injury from repetitive physical or mental motions.

Lately, I have been seeing more and more patients with muscle and tendon strains arising from poor circulation due to prolonged, repetitive motions at work. The most common example is probably carpal tunnel syndrome, which arises from the prolonged use of a computer keyboard. If you want to avoid suffering from such "repetitive strain syndrome" (RSI), remember not to forgo your ten-minute break lightly.

(b) Lunch break

Of course, the most important of these regular breaks is the one in the middle of the day — lunch break. Besides allowing ourselves a chance to disengage from work and retreat temporarily to the resting yin state, we are also acquiring vital substance from food during the lunch break. In order to accomplish both

> HABIT #49:
> Give yourself one full hour for lunch break so you can temporarily disengage from work and retreat to the resting yin state.

objectives, we need to give ourselves one full hour — don't hurry, slow down your pace, concentrate on the tastes, textures and aromas to promote good digestion (also discussed in Sect. 2-11).

(c) Overtime work

Then there is the ultimate break — the one at the end of the work day, which signifies the time we should be going home to get ready for the "other night job" of self-healing. Delaying this final break, as in the case of working overtime, although sometimes necessary, jeopardizes your chance to fully self-repair, which, in turn, jeopardizes your performance for the following days. Not only that, but working overtime can easily put your body into an energy debt situation, which can bring along a whole list of chronic health problems, including chronic fatigue, digestive problems, insomnia, etc. (see Sect. 3-1).

> HABIT #50:
> Keep overtime work to a minimum to avoid interrupting your "other night job" of self-healing.

As I have discussed previously (Sect. 3-2), you should keep overtime work at an absolute minimum and accept overtime work only if you have been building up a good surplus of vital essence through a healthy schedule of eating, work and rest. This may mean making choices about how much you want to work versus earn, negotiating with coworkers or family members for a better work schedule, or even re-examining your career and family goals so as to adjust to the needs of your health.

Sect. 5-8: Recharging throughout the year

(a) Winter dormancy

Just as many plants go into a dormant state in fall and winter to renew their energy for the following spring, many animals also enter a relative "dormant" state during the shorter and colder days of winter — it just does not seem as pronounced for us humans since, unlike frogs, snakes, bats, ground squirrels and bears, we do not hibernate and cease functioning. In reality, we ten d to spend less active hours outdoors, sleep longer, reduce our work hours and emphasize more on eating nutrient-rich foods. It may be just as well that a series of holidays clusters around this time of the year — Halloween (Harvest Festival), Thanksgiving, Hanukkah, Winter Solstice, Christmas, New Year, winter break (for college students), Martin Luther King Jr. Day, Lunar New Year, Mardi Gras, Valentine's Day, President's Day — most of them emphasize resting, eating and staying home with loved ones.

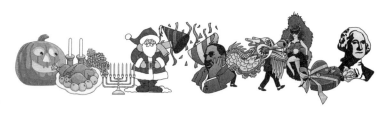
Do you think it is pure co-incident that so many holidays are packed within the winter months of November to February?

HABIT #51:
Allow your body for extra rest during the winter months in response to its need for a relative dormancy.

Biologically, we are simply responding to the colder temperature of winter, during which the pores of the skin close and sweating is reduced to prevent moisture loss, more food is consumed to build up an energy reserve to produce body heat, and physical activities are reduced to conserve energy and to avoid exposure to the outdoors. By allowing extra rest during the winter months, the body is able to focus its energy inward to heal while saving energy to support the anticipated growth and activity burst in the spring. During the winter months, one should be aware of these subtle needs of the body and not force it to work beyond its ability — or else it will become prone to illness during and after winter.

(b) Vacations

Whatever the season, however, we also need to take occasional breaks from our career, academic and family commitments — in other words, we need to occasionally turn from "doing for others" to "doing for ourselves". Two popular ways to achieve this goal are taking vacations and participating in hobbies.

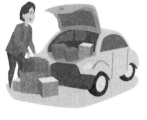

On your vacation, be sure to emphasize the relaxing and change of pace — don't let the packing and traveling overwhelm your trip.

A vacation can take the form of an elaborate two-week travel to Hawaii or a simple weekend camping trip at a nearby state park — it does not have to be luxurious or expensive as long as it provides a change of routine and surroundings, and a chance to relax and enjoy yourself in a restorative yin state. Therefore, while you are on vacation, be sure to take a comfortable pace and not worry about meeting a self-imposed tour schedule; be sure to focus on the sight and scenery and not worry about the responsibilities you left behind. Once you finish your journey of self-restoration, you will have fresh energy to return to your personal and career challenges.

(c) Hobbies

Again, the goal of participating in hobbies is to allow us a change of surroundings and to temporarily escape from our daily responsibilities and routines. You get to do something not because someone else wants it done but because you yourself want it done — to please yourself, to express yourself, to train yourself, or to challenge yourself. You are in your own world that you create for yourself.

Needless to say, hobbies are highly diverse and highly personalized according to the interests of each individual. For some, hobbies may be an artistic pursuit such as painting, music, sculpting, knitting or acting; while for others, hobbies may be a physical endeavor such as surfing, ballroom dancing, yoga or walking through the woods. Then there are those that focus on a specialized field of knowledge — classic cars restoration, gardening, model trains collection, video production, local history appreciation, bird watching.

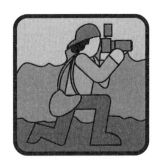

Hobbies do not have to be overly expensive or difficult. Try something you can enjoy without feeling burdened, like nature photography.

In any case, hobbies allow us to develop expertise and skills while simultaneously giving us a sense of personal fulfillment. Hobbies provide a link to the healing rhythm of yin and yang, of work and play, of self and others, and of giving and receiving. It is the balance of the two opposing phases of daily, weekly and seasonal life that gives us the sense of renewal and regeneration necessary for maintaining a healthy body and mind.

> HABIT #52:
> Give your body a chance for a change of pace and surrounding by taking vacations and participating in hobbies throughout the year.

CHAPTER 6
GOOD HEALTH HABITS

Sect. 6-1: The task ahead

Sect. 6-2: The complete list of good health habits

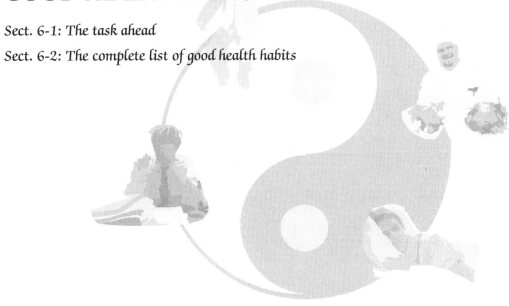

Sect. 6-1: The task ahead

So there you have it. You have learnt the secret of healthy living according to the theories of Chinese traditional medicine. You have the power of driving a smooth-running machine that can heal itself and stay out of major problems.

The only remaining job for you is to implement those health habits that we have discussed along the way — into practice. From now on, you ought to pay attention to your current living habits and begin to bring them in line with TCM practice. Use a pace that you feel most comfortable and, in time, you will be encouraged by the improvement of your health. At that time, you will be motivated to further accelerate the transition to the complete set of proper health habits.

Sect. 6-2: The complete list of good health habits

What I think will be useful is to make a complete list of proper TCM health habits below as your often-revisited reference. Go ahead and check off those habits that you are already practicing now. Then, once a week, return to review the list and check off more of the habits that you have newly adopted.

Your transition to a healthy way of life will be completed when you have checked off all the items in the list.

Good luck and enjoy living healthily!

☐ Habit #1: (Sect. 2-7, p. 46)

Eat well-balanced meals with a mix of grains, vegetables and meats, roughly in the ratio of 50%-25%-25%.

☐ Habit #2: (Sect. 2-7, p. 46)

Prepare meals from natural, unprocessed grains, vegetables and meats, instead of packaged, highly-processed ingredients.

☐ Habit #3: (Sect. 2-8, p. 47)

Eat a moderate amount of fruits after lunch and dinner to stimulate digestion, but avoid them in the morning.

☐ Habit #4: (Sect. 2-9, p. 49)

Drink a hot fluid, such as soup, seed-based nutritious drink, herbal tea or hot water before and after a meal to pre-heat and lubricate the digestive tract.

☐ Habit #5: (Sect. 2-10a, p. 51)

> *Avoid cold drinks and cold foods during regular meals; instead, heat them up or replace them with hot alternatives.*

☐ Habit #6: (Sect. 2-10a, p. 51)

> *Eat small amount of cold dessert occasionally for fun and only in a warm day.*

☐ Habit #7: (Sect. 2-10b, p. 52)

> *Always cook vegetables before eating to soften the plant tissue and to release the vitamins from the cell wall.*

☐ Habit #8: (Sect. 2-10c, p. 54)

> *Avoid eating direct-fire and deep-fried foods in regular meals.*

☐ Habit #9: (Sect. 2-10d, p. 55)

> *Stay away from spicy foods to prevent exposing your internal organs from overstimulation.*

☐ Habit #10: (Sect. 2-10e, p. 56)

> *Avoid the use of garlic in cooking and never ingest garlic to prevent over-stimulating the body.*

☐ Habit #11: (Sect. 2-10f, p. 58)

> *Avoid eating overly sweetened, packaged foods to prevent from overworking the pancreas, liver and kidney.*

☐ Habit #12: (Sect. 2-10g, p. 60)

> *Avoid taking supplements as a source of nutrients — instead, obtain nutrients from natural sources.*

☐ Habit #13: (Sect. 2-10h, p. 62)

> *Eliminate the need to use stimulants by identifying and correcting the faulty living habits that are causing your health problems.*

☐ Habit #14: (Sect. 2-11, p. 64)

> *Pay equal attention to your work and eating habits — carefully plan for three well-balanced meals every day at regular, predictable times.*

☐ Habit #15: (Sect. 2-11a, p. 65)

> *For breakfast, avoid coffee, juice and fruit, but fill your stomach to 100% capacity with hot, easy-to-digest, semi-liquid food selections.*

☐ Habit #16: (Sect. 2-11b, p. 66)

> *Eat lunch in a pleasant environment with a relaxed pace and finish with a small piece of fruit.*

☐ Habit #17: (Sect. 2-11c, p. 67)

> *Eat dinner at a fixed, predictable time, two to three hours before sleep, and avoid snacking before dinner time.*

☐ Habit #18: (Sect. 2-11c, p. 68)

> *Eat a piece of fruit for dessert to enhance digestion and to avoid taking in unnecessary amount of sugar.*

☐ Habit #19: (Sect. 2-12, p. 70)

> *Avoid cooking by intense heat (such as barbecue, grilling, charbroiling and deep frying) and the use of heavy flavoring (such as thick dressings, overly salty or sweet sauces, hot sauce and spices).*

☐ Habit #20: (Sect. 2-12c, p. 75)

Use proper cooking methods, such as water-cooking, steaming and stir-frying, to bring out the natural flavors while preserving the nutrition and moisture content of food.

☐ Habit #21: (Sect. 2-13, p. 77)

Take appropriate measures when eating out to maintain good eating habits and to avoid foods that harm our health.

☐ Habit #22: (Sect. 3-1, p. 91)

Pay close attention to your body for signs of energy debt. When they occur, instead of just reaching into the drug cabinet for quick fixes of the symptoms, immediately make adjustments to your living habits to ease the energy debt crisis.

☐ Habit #23: (Sect. 3-2a, p. 93)

In order to utilize your energy more cost-effectively, avoid extending daytime work activities into late evening with better time management.

☐ Habit #24: (Sect. 3-2a, p. 93)

Avoid late-night entertainments which prevent the body from receiving proper rest when rest is needed

☐ Habit #25: (Sect. 3-2b, p. 95 and Sect. 5-7a, p. 151)

Take a ten-minute break for every two hours of work in order (1) to allow the body's recharging process to catch up with energy spending, and (2) to avoid injury from repetitive physical or mental motions.

☐ Habit #26: (Sect. 3-3 p. 97)

Do not overexert yourself with strenuous exercise if you have a full-time workload or if the time has already passed 6 P.M.

☐ Habit #27: (Sect. 3-3, p. 98)

> *Replace strenuous exercises with practical exercises around the house or gentle exercises that do not overtax your body.*

☐ Habit #28: (Sect. 3-4, p.100)

> *Set limit to the amount of over-stimulating entertainments you engage in, particularly those that occur during the evening hours.*

☐ Habit #29: (Sect. 3-4, p. 101)

> *Try to ease yourself out of intense mental or emotional state by using the techniques of meditation and physical release.*

☐ Habit #30: (Sect. 3-5a, p. 104)

> *During transition time between seasons, bring a jacket and a hat with you and, with no hesitation, wear them at the first sign of chill.*

☐ Habit #31: (Sect. 3-5a, p. 105)

> *Prevent you hair, clothes and shoes from getting wet from rain, and if they do, dry or change them at the earliest possible instant.*

☐ Habit #32: (Sect. 3-5a, p. 105)

> *Watch out for "wind chill": protect your head and shoulder from breezes, and stay away from cold draft near open window.*

☐ Habit #33: (Sect. 3-5b, p. 106)

> *Avoid direct contact with cold or damp surfaces — use a layer of insulation if necessary.*

☐ Habit #34: (Sect. 3-5c, p. 106)

> *Avoid breathing in dry or damp air — use a humidifier or dehumidifier to improve the air in such conditions.*

☐ Habit #35: (Sect. 3-5d, p. 107)

> *Do not wash your hair every time you shower and, when you do, blow-dry it immediately after washing.*

☐ Habit #36: (Sect. 3-5d, p. 108)

> *Take warm shower in the evening before bed time instead of in the morning immediately after rising from bed.*

☐ Habit #37: (Sect. 3-5e, p. 110)

> *In winter, do not set the heater too high but rely on jacket and comforter to keep warm; in summer, do not set the air conditioner too low, but allow light sweating to keep cool.*

☐ Habit #38: (Sect. 3-5e, p. 111)

> *In summer, when entering an area with strong air conditioning, immediately wipe off your sweat and put on a jacket; in winter, put on extra layers before stepping out to the cold outdoors, and take shelter to allow time for your body to adjust.*

☐ Habit #39: (Sect. 3-5f, p. 111)

> *Do not take food or drinks that have been chilled with ice so that your body does not have to waste energy to heat them up.*

☐ Habit #40: (Sect. 4-2, p. 120)

> *Learn and practice non-movement-style chi gong for 15 minutes before bed time to relax the mind and body into peaceful sleep.*

☐ Habit #41: (Sect. 4-3, p. 123)

> *If you are in healthy condition and prefer to move around while exercising, learn and practice a version of moving-style chi gong that is suitable for you.*

☐ Habit #42: (Sect. 4-4, p. 127)

> *Practice acupressure and reflexology techniques at home as instructed by your TCM practitioner in order to promote healing by enhancing chi flow.*

☐ Habit #43: (Sect. 5-5, p.147)

> *Go to bed promptly at 10:30 P.M. every night so that you will be in deep sleep by 11:00 P.M. for the gall bladder fortified chi (11 P.M. - 1 A.M.) and liver fortified chi (1 A.M. - 3A.M.).*

☐ Habit #44: (Sect. 5-5, p. 148)

> *Give yourself 8 hours of sleep so your body has sufficient time to fully self-regenerate.*

☐ Habit #45: (Sect. 5-6, p. 148)

> *Go to bed at the same time every night so that your body can anticipate the coming yin state and naturally fall asleep.*

☐ Habit #46: (Sect. 5-6, p. 149)

> *Allow two to three hours between the end of dinner and the beginning of bedtime so your digestive system can rest when you sleep.*

☐ Habit #47: (Sect. 5-6, p. 149)

> *Prepare yourself to sleep by doing something that slows down your pace and, of course, do not over-stimulate yourself with vigorous exercise or high-power entertainment.*

☐ Habit #48: (Sect. 5-6, p. 150)

> *Make you sleeping environment comfortable — do not overheat or overcool the bedroom and do not allow cold draft near your bed.*

☐ Habit #49: (Sect. 5-7b, p. 151)

> *Give yourself one full hour for lunch break so you can temporarily disengage from work and retreat to the resting yin state.*

☐ Habit #50: (Sect. 5-7c, p. 152)

> *Keep overtime work to a minimum to avoid interrupting your "other night job" of self-healing.*

☐ Habit #51: (Sect. 5-8a, p. 153)

> *Allow your body for extra rest during the winter months in response to its need for a relative dormancy.*

☐ Habit #52: (Sect. 5-8c, p. 155)

> *Give your body a chance for a change of pace and surrounding by taking vacations and participating in hobbies throughout the year.*

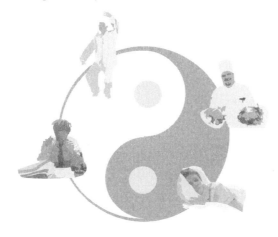

166

INDEX

A

Acupoints, 17
  in acupressure, 124
Acupressure
  as a chi-enhancing therapy, 124
  direct-pressure method, 124
  gentle-touch method, 125
  when and how to practice, 128
Acupuncture, 17
  as a chi-enhancing therapy, 124
  basis of, 17
Adrenal cortex
  adrenocorticosteroids from, 88
  stress hormones of, 20, 88
Adrenocorticosteroids, 88
  as immunosuppressant, 88
AIDS
  Karposi's sarcoma due to, 21
Air conditioning system
  highly-contrasting indoor and outdoor temperatures due to, 109
  proper setting in summer, 110
Airline operation
  versus human body, 130
Alcohol
  liver cirrhosis due to, 37
  negative emotions and, 89
  as stimulant, 60
  stomach bleeding due to, 32
Alzheimer's Disease
  due to amyloid-beta protein accumulation, 136
  liver and, 136
Ammonia
  conversion into urea, 135
  origin of, 135
Amyloid-beta protein
  misfolded
    Alzheimer's Disease and, 136
    liver and, 136
    Parkinson's Disease and, 136
Amylose, 30
Anemia
  due to failure to recycle iron from hemoglobin, 139
Anger
  due to energy debt, 89
  liver fire due to, 144
  due to liver stagnation, 144
Antioxidants
  for cleaning unreacted ROS, 142
Anxiety
  disorder
    due to imaginary threats, 101
  due to energy debt, 89
Appetite
  suppression of
    due to snacking, 67
Artificial sweeteners
  harmful effects to liver and kidney, 58
Atherosclerosis
  due to failure to regulate cholesterol by liver, 139

B

Balance
  between active and resting states, 23
  between births and deaths, 13
  between hot and cold energetic properties, 69
  between sun and rain, 13
  of the three food types, 43
  between vital substance and vital force, 14, 22
Bank account
  versus fuel tank of body, 14
BBQ, 53

Bicarbonate
　in pancreatic juice, 35
Bile, 35
　bile salt in, 35
　　as detergent, 35
　bilirubin and, 135
　for excretion of organic wastes, 136
　from gall bladder, 35
　from liver, 36
　organic wastes in, 142
　versus urine, 136
Bile canaliculi, 135
Bile duct
　for excretion of bilirubin, 135
Bilirubin, 135
　bile and, 135
　elimination of, by liver, 135
Blood
　into liver, 140
Blood flow
　of liver versus heart, 138
　through hepatic sinusoids, 143
Blood glucose
　diabetes and, 37
　overly sweetened foods and, 58
　stress hormones and, 88
Blood pressure
　in portal vein versus hepatic vein, 143
　stress hormones and, 88, 144
Body functions
　overheating of, due to "hot" food, 69
　slowing down of, due to "cold" food, 69
Body temperature
　teeth and, 29
Brain
　diseases
　　liver and, 136
　stimulants and, 61
Breakfast, 65
　food choices for, 65
　losing weight and, 65
　metabolic rate and, 65
Breaks. *See* Rest
Breast tumor
　due to liver failure, 137
Breathing
　dry or damp air
　　heat loss due to, 106
Business investment
　versus digestion, 27

C

Caffeine
　dehydration due to, 61
　as stimulant, 60
Calcium carbonate
　as calcium pills, 48
Calcium chondroitin sulfate, 49
Calcium pills
　inefficiency of, 48
Cancer
　in AIDS patients, 21
　cytotoxic T-cells and, 21
　direct cause of, 21
　due to DNA damages, 21
　immune system and, 20, 21
　indirect cause of, 21
　due to mutagens, 21
　natural killer cells and, 21
　rest and, 20
　of stomach, aftermath of, 33
　due to stress, 20
Capsaicin
　and pain sensation, 56
　versus MSG, 55
　as a neurotoxin, 55
　in spicy foods, 55
Car
　versus human body. *See* Human body: versus car
　problems, fixing, 2

Carbohydrates, 29
Carpal tunnel syndrome
   due to inadequate rest, 151
Cellulose. *See* Fibers
Cell wall
   cellulose in, 39
   nutrients within, 29
Chi, 16
   blockage, 17
      diseases due to, 17, 105
      fortified chi and, 132
      due to wind chill, 105
   fortified current, 132
      liver and, 147
   versus steam, 17
Chi-enhancing exercise. *See* Chi gong
Chi-enhancing therapies, 124
   acupressure as, 124
   acupuncture as, 124
   reflexology as, 125
   when and how to practice, 128
Chi gong
   as light exercise, 98
   as meditation, 102, 119
   build up of chi circulation, 119
   class, 121
   martial-art-style, 123
      for self-defense, competition and exhibition, 123
   moving-style, 122
      for health maintenance, 123
      Tai Chi as, 122
      Tai Chi Chuan as, 123
   non-movement-style, 117
      advantages of, 120
      best time to practice, 120
      for health building, 123
   physical experience during, 119
   principles of, 117
   to promote sleep, 149
   versus regular exercises, 113, 117
   sitting posture, 119
   standing pose, 119
   when to practice, 127
Chinese herbal medicine
   basic principle of, 69
Cholesterol
   elimination through bile, 136
   plaques in arterial wall, 139
      thrombosis and, 139
Chondroitin sulfate, 49
Chronic fatigue. *See* Fatigue: chronic
Chyme, 34
   neutralization of, 35
Cigarette
   diseases due to, 61
   negative emotions and, 89
   as stimulant, 60
Circadian rhythm
   sleep and, 149
Circulatory system
   liver and, 138
Coffee
   as stimulant, 61
   fatigue and, 84
   seed-based drinks to replace, 66
Cold desserts, 51
Cold drinks
   diseases due to, 51
   inhibition on digestion by, 50
   peristalsis and, 50
   stomach and, 51
Cold or damp conditions
   due to direct contact, 106
   due to weather conditions, 103
Colon cancer
   peristalsis and, 40
Compulsive thinking
   anxiety disorder due to, 101
   depression due to, 101
   as imaginary threat, 100
   meditation for, 101
   physical release for, 101

Confucianism, 12
Confucius, 12
Constipation
  cause of, 39
  due to energy debt, 85
  hemorrhoid due to, 39
  due to liver stagnation, 144
  peristalsis and, 39
Contact
  with cold or damp surfaces
    heat loss due to, 106
Cooking
  by intense heat
    reasons to avoid, 70
  methods
    criteria for proper, 70
  purpose of, 68
  to neutralize energetic properties
    of foods, 68
Cortisol
  as stress hormone, 20
  as immunosuppressant, 20
Coughing
  due to "cold" food, 69
Curd regurgitation
  due to cold milk, 51
Cytotoxic T-cells
  cancer and, 21

D

Dampness, 41
Daoism. *See* Taoism
Dehumidifier
  for damp air, 106
Dehydration
  due to caffeine, 61
  state of
    due to direct-fire or deep-fried
      foods, 54
Denaturation of protein, 32
  due to hydrochloric acid, 32

Depression
  due to imaginary threats, 101
Desserts
  after dinner, 68
  cold, 51
Detergent
  for lipid digestion, 35
Detoxification
  in liver, 135, 141
Diabetes
  blood glucose and, 37
  insulin and, 35
  liver and, 134
  due to overly sweetened foods, 58
  pancreas and, 35
  type II
    as a liver-related disease, 134
Diarrhea
  due to energy debt, 85
Diet
  common notion of healthy, 42
  TCM concept of healthy, 43
  vegetarian, 44
    protein deficiency and, 45
    sedentary lifestyle and, 45
Dietary supplements
  common rationale for taking, 59
  kidney and, 60
  liver and, 60
  versus natural food sources, 59
  spleen and, 60
Digestion
  versus business investment, 27
  downward spiral of poor, 28
  goal of, 29
  as investment of energy, 27
  preparation for a new round of, 67
  in small intestine, 36
Digestive enzymes
  depletion due to snacking, 67
  inhibition due to cold drinks, 50

as molecular scissors, 30
water and temperature for, 48
Digestive system
gearing up for meal by, 67
good health and, 28
liver and, 134
problems of
due to energy debt, 85
stunning of
by cold drinks, 50
Dinner
timing relative to sleep, 67
Discomfort
versus disease, 10
Diseases
acute
examples of, 2
causes of, 6
chi blockage as, 17
chronic
energy acquisition and, 28
examples of, 2
kidney functions and, 15
versus discomfort, 10
in modern society, 2
due to protein deficiency, 45
due to smoking, 61
theories of, 4
DNA damages
cancer due to, 21
Downward spiral of poor digestion, 28
Driness
in membranes, due to "hot" food, 69
Drip-delivery system
in psychological study of the mind, 117
Drug metabolism pathway, 141
Drugs. *See also* Recreational drug
elimination through bile, 136
Duodenum, 34
digestive juices in, 35
ulcer of, 35

E

Eating out
practical tips for, 76
Edginess
due to energy debt, 89
Electric radiator
for warming a room, 110
Emotions
extreme
liver fire due to, 144
due to liver stagnation, 144
as indicator of body's energy state, 89
negative
due to energy debt, 89
Emulsification
of lipids, 35
Endocrine system
liver and, in hormone regulation, 137
Endometriosis
due to liver failure, 137
Endorphins
during strenuous exercise, 96
Energetic properties of food, 68
Chinese herbal medicine and, 69
neutralizing, with cooking, 68
ginger root for, 71, 72, 74, 75
green onion for, 75
Energetic state of body, 69
Chinese herbal medicine, 69
neutralizing with herbs and foods, 69
Energy
debt, 83
versus a computer without power, 85
signs of, 83
chronic fatigue as, 84
digestive problems, 85
hot flashes as, 87
insomnia as, 86
muscle and tendon injuries as, 88
negative emotions as, 89
return of old symptoms as, 90

weak immune system as, 88
weight gain as, 90
flow, 16
as a limited resource, 82
savings
versus savings in bank account, 15
utilization of, 14
Entertainment
violent, scary or high-energy
loss of vital force and, 100
Erythrocytes. *See* Red blood cells
Escherichia coli
in intestine, 38
Esophagus, 31
windpipe, relative to, 31
Estrogen
abnormal growth of reproductive tissues and, 137
as mitogen, 137
regulation of, by liver, 137
Euphoria
due to strenuous exercise, 96
Excretory system
excretion of urine by, 135
liver and, 135
Exercise
benefits of, 114
drawback of, 115
for the sick and injured, 117
gentle, 98
chi gong as, 98
practical, 97
strenuous
alternatives to, 97
common view about, 96
reasons to avoid, 97
who should avoid, 96
versus chi gong, 117
Eye
fatigue
as sign of liver failure, 136

due to liver stagnation, 144

F

Fat
converted from excess glucose, 58
Fatigue
chronic
coffee and, 84
due to energy debt, 84
due to poor energy acquisition, 28
temporary, 84
Fear
due to energy debt, 89
Ferritin
storage in and release from liver, 139
Fibers, 39
indigestibility of, 39
peristalsis and, 39
in plant cell wall, 39
Fibromyalgia
due to poor energy acquisition, 28
Fight-or-flight response, 99
due to compulsive thinking, 100
due to dangerous situations, 99
due to imaginary threats, 99
due to intense emotion, 100
due to violent and scary entertainment, 100
negative effects of, 99
Finger stick
for reflexology, 127
Flight
Asia-bound versus America-bound, 146
Flu. *See* Influenza
Food choices
for breakfast, 65
for dinner, 68
for lunch, 66
in potlucks, 77
when eating out, 77

Foods
　deep-fried, 53
　direct-fire, 53
　overly sweetened, 57
　　diabetes due to, 58
　　liver and, 58
　　obesity due to, 58
　　pancreas and, 58
　　sugar from, 58
　packaged, 57
　　fortified vitamins in, 58
　raw, 52
　spicy, 54
　　internal organs and, 55
　　as a measure of toughness, 54
Food therapy, 49
Food types
　proportions of, 46
　three major, 43
Fruit concentrate
　as pre-meal hot fluid, 50
Fruits
　as desserts after dinner, 68
　benefits of, 47
　purging effect of, 47
　when to avoid eating, 47
　when to eat, 47
Frustration
　due to energy debt, 89
Fuel tank of body
　versus bank account, 14

G

Gall bladder
　bile from, 35
　functions of, 36
　liver and, 147
　removal of,, 36
Gallstones
　as a liver-related disease, 134
　cause of, 142

Garlic, 56
　harmful effects of, 56
　insomnia due to, 56
　proper use for cooking, 56
　as a stimulant, 56
Gas (intestinal). *See* Intestinal gas
Gastric bypass, 33
Gastric glands, 31
Gastric juice, 34
Ginger root
　for neutralizing cool property of fish, 75
　for neutralizing cool property of vegetables, 70, 71
Glucagon
　in blood glucose regulation, 37
Glucocorticoids
　blood vessel constriction due to, 144
Glucosamine, 49
Glycogen, 37
Grains
　as a major food type, 43
Gravy
　after stir-frying, 75
Green onion
　to neutralize warm property of meats, 75

H

Hair washing
　best time for, 107
　blow-dryer and, 108
　frequency of, 107
　minimizing time of exposure during, 107
Healing and the Mind
　by Bill Moyer, 121
Health
　good
　　conventional ideas of, 9
　　digestive system and, 28
　　TCM interpretation of, 11, 22
Health habits, 7

good, 7, 23
  four strategies for, 23
Health problems. *See also* Diseases
  quick fixes to, 3
Heart
  attack
    liver and, 139
  hot flash and, 87
  spicy foods and, 55
Heartburn, 31
  due to energy debt, 85
Heating system
  highly-contrasting indoor and outdoor temperatures due to, 109
  proper setting in winter, 110
Heat loss from human body, 102
  due to breathing dry or damp air, 106
  due to cold and damp conditions, 103
  due to cold drinks and food, 111
  due to contact with cold surface, 106
  due to faulty washing habits, 107
  versus heat loss from home, 103
  due to highly-contrasting indoor and outdoor temperatures, 109
  preventing, 103
Helicobacter pylori, 32
Hemoglobin
  recycling of iron in, by liver, 139
Hemorrhoid, 39
  due to constipation, 39
  prevention of, 40
Hepatic sinusoids, 135
Highly-contrasting indoor and outdoor temperatures
  avoiding, at home, 110
  heat loss due to, 109
  precautions, at public places, 110
Hobbies, 154
Holidays
  during winter months, 153
Homeostasis, 36

Hormones
  clearance of, by liver, 137
Hot flash
  due to energy debt, 87
  heart and, 87
  due to phantom flame, 87
Hot fluids
  for absorbable calcium, 49
  for soluble nutrients, 48
  for lubrication and pre-warming, 48
  when eating out, 76
Human body
  versus airline operation, 130
  theory of yin-and-yang and, 14
  versus car
    as machines, 1
    in energy utilization, 14
    in quick fixes, 3
  versus self-healing machine, 18
  versus steam engine, 16
Humidifier
  for dry air, 106
Hydrochloric acid, 31
  in denaturation of proteins, 32
  in killing of microbes, 32
  in pepsin activation, 33

I

Ice water
  as a cold drink, 50
  when eating out, 76
Immune system
  cancer and, 21
  mobilization by Kupffer cells in liver, 138
  sleep and, 19
  stress and, 21
  stress hormones and, 20
  weakened
    due to energy debt, 88

Indigestion
  due to cold drinks, 51
  due to energy debt, 85
  due to lack of fluid, 48
  due to liver stagnation, 144
Infertility
  due to liver failure, 137
Inflammation
  due to "hot" food, 69
Influenza, **5**
  direct cause of, 6
  due to energy debt, 88
  due to highly-contrasting indoor and outdoor temperatures, 109
  indirect cause of, 6
  sleep and, 6, 19
  virus, 5
  weather and, 6
Injury
  of muscles and tendons
    as sign of energy debt, 89
    due to energy debt, 89
  rest and, 20
Insomnia
  due to liver stagnation, 144
  due to energy debt, 86
  melatonin and, 87
  paradox of, 86
  relief from, with chi gong, 120
  sleeping pill and, 87
  due to stimulatory effect of garlic, 56
  tranquilizer and, 87
Insulin
  blood glucose and, 37
  chronic exposure to elevated level of, 58
  diabetes and, 35
  liver and, 37
  resistance, 58
Intense emotion
  anxiety disorder due to, 101
  depression due to, 101
  as imaginary threat, 100
  meditation for, 101
  physical release for, 101
Intestinal gas
  due to cold drinks, 51
  due to energy debt, 85
Iron
  recovery from dead red blood cells by liver, 139
Irritability
  due to liver stagnation, 144

J

Jaundice
  due to bilirubin, 136
  as a liver-related disease, 134
Jet stream
  of liver, 147
  of gall bladder, 147
  over the Pacific Ocean, 147
Joints
  ache, due to "hot" food, 69

K

Karposi's sarcoma
  due to AIDS, 21
Kidney
  dietary supplements and, 60
  excretion of urine by, 135
  spicy foods and, 55
  weight gain and, 90
Kung Fu
  as martial-art-style chi gong, 123
Kupffer cells
  as defense against invaders, 137, 141
  co-ordination with helper T-lymphocytes, 138
  mobilization of immune system by, 138
  recycling of red blood cells by, 139

L

Laptop computer
  recharging battery of
    versus taking daytime rests, 95
Large intestine
  bacteria in, 38
  processing of indigestible waste in, 38
Laws of heredity
  as hypotheses with unknown biochemical basis, 18
Lipids, 29
  digestion of, 35
  emulsification of, 35
Liver, 36
  abnormal growth in reproductive tissues and, 137
  artificial sweeteners and, 58
  as an emergency blood reservoir, 138
  blood flow through, 138
    resistance to, 143
  blood from intestine into, 140
  blood glucose regulation by, 37
  circulatory system and, 138
  cirrhosis, 38
    due to alcohol, 37, 61
    due to toxins, 141
    resistance to blood flow due to, 143
  congestion
    due to stress, 145
  as a dam against flooding of nutrients, 36
  desensitization to insulin of, 58
  detoxification in, 135, 141
  dietary supplements and, 60
  digestive system and, 134
  elimination of toxins and wastes, 136, 141
  emotional stress and, 144
  endocrine system and, 137
  excretory system and, 135
  eyes and, 136
  fire, 144
  as first-line defense, 137
  fortified chi and, 147
  functions of, in TCM, 41
  gall bladder and, 147
  immune system and, 137
  nervous system and, 136
  as origin of all diseases, 133
  overly sweetened foods and, 58
  reactive oxygen species in, 142
  recycling of red blood cells by, 139
  regeneration, 146
  regulation of cholesterol by, 139
  reproductive system and, 137
  spicy foods and, 55
  stagnation, 144
  storage of glucose in, 58
  storage, synthesis and breaking down of biochemicals by, 37
  stress and, 144
  weight gain and, 90
Living organism
  definition of, 14
Lunch, 66, 151
  food selections, 66
Lunch break, 151
Lung congestion
  due to chi blockage, 105
Lymph
  formation in liver, 135

M

Mealtimes
  regular
    common rationale of missing, 63
    planning for, 64
    reasons for, 64
    reasons for fixing, 67
    rule of, 63
Meats

cooking, 73
  by more elaborated methods, 73
  by steaming, 73
  by stir-frying, 74
  as a major food type, 44
  marinating before cooking, 73
Meditation, 102
  chi gong as, 102
  for compulsory thinking, 102
  for intense emotion, 102
Melatonin
  insomnia and, 87
Mendel, Gregor, 18
Menstruation
  difficulty in, due to "cold" food, 69
  excessive flow in
    due to liver failure, 137
  irregular
    due to liver failure, 137
  lack of flow
    due to liver failure, 137
  seepage of
    due to poor energy acquisition, 28
Meridian clock, 132
  as schedule of chi focus, 133
Meridians, 16
  clogging of
    due to dampness, 42
    due to excess nutrients, 60
  lung-related, 132
  patterns of, 125
  properties of, 17
Metabolic rate
  breakfast and, 65
  excessive, due to "hot" food, 69
Microbes
  hydrochloric acid and, 32
Mind
  effect on involuntary functions, 118
    neuroendocrine connection and, 118
  exercise of
    chi gong as, 119

  power over body, 117
    as placebo effect, 118
    as psychological effect, 118
    psychological study of, 117
    versus wishful thinking, 118
Minerals, 29
Moyer, Bill
  Healing and the Mind by, 121
MSG
  versus capsaicin, 55
Mucus
  accumulation in respiratory tract, due to "cold" food, 69
  from large intestine, 38
  on stomach wall, 31
Muscle aches
  due to chi blockage, 105
Mutagens
  cancer due to, 21

N

Natural killer cells, 21
Negative emotions. *See* Emotions: negative
Nervous system
  liver and, 136
Neuroendocrine connection
  as mind-body connection, 118
Night jobs
  decision to accept, 93
Nightlife activities
  alternatives to, 94
  harmful effect of, 94
Night shift
  as nighttime activities, 93
Night sweat. *See* Hot flash
Nighttime activities
  extra overhead cost for, 92
  for entertainment, 94
  versus rowing a canoe against the current, 93

Nutrients, 29
  balancing of, by liver, 134
  in blood entering liver, 140

O

Obesity
  due to overly sweetened foods, 58
  gastric bypass for, 33
Oral cavity, 29
  saliva in, 30
  salivary amylase in, 30
  starch digestion in, 30
Organic wastes
  in bile, 142
Ovarian cyst
  due to liver failure, 137
Over-exercising
  common reason for, 95
Overtime work, 152
  as nighttime activities, 93

P

Pain
  lower back
    due to depletion of kidney functions, 16
  shoulder and back
    self-healing and, 19
Pancreas, 35
  diabetes and, 35
  overly sweetened foods and, 58
  pancreatic juice from, 35
Pancreatic juice, 35
  bicarbonate in, 35
  digestive enzymes in, 35
Parkinson's Disease
  liver and, 136
Pasta
  cooking, 71
Pathogens
  food-borne, 141

Pepsin
  activation of, 33
    hydrochloric acid and, 33
Peptic ulcers, 35
Peristalsis, 34
  cold drinks and, 50
  colon cancer and, 40
  constipation and, 39
  fibers and, 39
Peroxides
  in liver, 141
Phantom flame (TCM)
  due to chronic fatigue, 85
Physical release, 102
  for compulsory thinking, 101
  for intense emotion, 101
Placebo effect
  versus mind over body, 118
Poor concentration
  due to poor energy acquisition, 28
Potlucks
  eating healthily in, 77
Premenstrual syndrome (PMS)
  due to liver failure, 137
Progesterone
  regulation of, by liver, 137
Proneness to injury
  due to energy debt, 89
Prostate enlargement
  due to liver failure, 137
Protein deficiency
  diseases due to, 45
Proteins, 29
  denaturation of, 32
    due to hydrochloric acid, 32
  plant versus animal, 44, 45
Psychological effect
  versus mind over body, 118
Pushing hands
  as a two-person version of Tai Chi Chuan, 123

Q

Qi. *See* Chi
Qigong. *See* Chi gong

R

Reactive oxygen species (ROS)
  cell damage by, 142
  in liver, 142
Recreational drug
  negative emotions and, 89
  semantic ambiguity of, 62
  as stimulant, 61
Red blood cells
  recycling of, by liver, 139
Reflexology, 125
  as a chi-enhancing therapy, 125
  charts, 126
  finger stick for, 126, 127
  pain sensation during, 126
  river rocks for, 127
  walnut for, 127
  when and how to practice, 128
Repetitive strain syndrome (RSI)
  due to inadequate rest, 151
Reproductive system
  liver and, 137
Resentment
  due to energy debt, 89
Rest
  from career and commitments, 154
  during daytime, 150
    activities for, 151
    frequency of, 95, 151
    reason for, 95
    as recharging process, 95
  during winter months, 153
  inadequate, 19, 95
    energy debt and, 95
  injury and, 20
  during nighttime, 131
  self-healing and, 19
  versus work, 131
Restless leg syndrome
  due to poor energy acquisition, 28
Return of old symptoms
  due to energy debt, 90
Rice
  cooking with rice cooker, 71
River rocks
  for reflexology, 127
Rowing a canoe
  against current
    versus nighttime activities, 93

S

Salad
  as raw foods, 52
Saliva, 30
Salivary amylase, 30
Salivary glands, 30
Savings, 15
  equation of, 26, 82
  purpose of, 15
Seed-based drinks, 49
  as replacement for coffee, 66
Self-healing
  versus aircraft maintenance, 19
  energy debt and, 88
  error messages during, 86
  exercise in evening and, 97
  importance of, 18
  night job of, 131
  rest and, 19
  during resting state, 19, 86
  shoulder and back pain and, 19
Showers (washing)
  best time in a day for, 108
  hot, 108
Sinus infection
  due to chi blockage, 105

Siu Lin Gong
  as martial-art-style chi gong, 123
Sleep
  best time to, 132, 148
  circadian rhythm and, 149
  environment, 150
  exercising in evening and, 97
  fortified chi and, 147
  healthy, 150
  immune system and, 19
  influenza and, 6, 19
  tips for good-quality, 148
Sleep disorder
  due to energy debt, 86
Sleeping pill
  insomnia and, 87
Slow down
  of body functions, due to "cold food", 69
Small intestine
  absorption in, 36
  digestion in, 36
  duodenum of, 34
Smoking. See Cigarette
Snacks
  reason not to eat, 67
  when not to, 67
Sole
  for reflexology, 125
Soup
  for calcium, 49
Spasm
  of nerves, due to "hot" food, 69
Spleen
  chi, 41
  dietary supplements and, 60
  as a distilling organ, 41
  failure of, due to "cold food", 69
  functions of, in TCM, 41
  as pancreas, in TCM, 41
  spraying of vital substance by, 41

Stagnation
  due to "cold" food, 69
  of liver, 144
Starch
  digestion in oral cavity, 30
Steam
  versus chi, 17
Steam engine
  versus human body, 16
Steaming
  benefits of, 73
  meats, 73
Steroid hormones
  elimination through bile, 136
Stimulants, 60
  brain and, 61
  common rationale for using, 62
  solution to stop using, 62
Stir-frying
  benefits of, 72
  meats, 74
  vegetables, 72
Stomach, 31
  acid, 31
  bleeding, 32
    alcohol and, 32
  cancer, aftermath of, 33
  chi, 51
  cold
    due to energy debt, 85
  cold drinks and, 51
  as cooking pot, 40
  function of, 33
  function of, in TCM, 40
  gastric bypass in, 33
  gastric glands in, 31
  gastric juice in, 34
  hydrochloric acid in, 31
  mucus in, 31
  sphincters, 31
  surgery for weight loss, 33

ulcer, 32
upset
  due to cold drinks, 51
wall, 31
  virus entry through, 32
Strains
  of muscle and tendons
    due to inadequate rest, 151
Stress
  cancer due to, 20
  decline of liver functions due to, 144
  immune system and, 21
  liver congestion due to, 145
  liver fire due to, 144
  due to liver stagnation, 144
  as physiological issue, 145
  relief from, with chi gong, 120
  stomach ulcer due to, 32
Stress hormones
  blood vessel constriction due to, 144
  immune system and, 20
Stroke
  liver and, 139
Sugar
  from overly sweetened foods, 58
  suitable uses of, 59
Superoxide
  in liver, 142

T

Tai Chi, 122
  as moving-style chi gong, 122
  balance and concentration in, 122
Tai Chi Chuan
  as moving-style chi gong, 123
  pushing hands as a form of, 123
Taoism, 12
TCM concepts
  challenges in explaining, 7
Tea
  as pre-meal hot fluid, 50
Teeth, 29
  body temperature and, 30
  in mammals, 29
  in reptiles, 30
Tendinitis
  due to chi blockage, 105
  due to depletion of kidney functions, 16
Testosterone
  abnormal growth in reproductive tissues and, 137
  as mitogen, 137
Thirst
  constant
    due to liver stagnation, 144
Thrombosis
  liver and, 139
Tongue, 29
Toxic chemicals
  ammonia as, 135
  bilirubin as, 135
  collected by liver cells, 141
  elimination by liver, 135
Traditional Chinese medicine. *See* TCM
Tranquilizer
  insomnia and, 87
Tui Na. *See* Acupressure

U

Urea
  conversion from ammonia, 135
  excretion through urine, 135
Uterine fibroid
  due to liver failure, 137

V

Vacations, 154
Vegetables
  cooking of
    benefits of, 52

common objections to, 53
  by stir-frying, 72
  by water cooking, 71
as a major food type, 43
for prevention of hemorrhoid, 40
purpose of eating, 39, 40
for vitamins, 40
Vegetarian diet. *See* Diet: vegetarian
Vital essence, 15
  depletion of, 15
  equation of, 26, 82
Vital force, 14
  conserving
    goal of, 82
Vital substance, 14
  mist of, 41
Vitamins, 29
  from bacteria in intestine, 38
  within cell wall of vegetables, 52
  fortified in packaged foods, 58
  from vegetables, 40

W

Walnut
  for reflexology, 127
Warring States period, 11
Water
  ice, 50
  as pre-meal hot fluid, 50
Water cooking
  vegetables, 71
Weapon manipulation
  as martial-art-style chi gong, 123
Weather
  fluctuating, 104
    influenza due to, 104
  influenza and, 6
Weight gain
  as a dietary problem, 90
  due to energy debt, 90

versus a home without cleaning, 91
  kidney and, 90
  liver and, 90
Weight loss
  breakfast and, 65
  gastric bypass for, 34
Wind chill (in TCM), 105
  chi blockage due to, 105
  prevention against, 105
Windpipe
  esophagus, relative to, 31
Winter dormancy, 153

Y

Yin and yang, 13
  theory of, 11
    human body and, 14

Z

Zhou Dynasty, 11
Zone therapy. *See* Reflexology